Reader Reviews

This book should be required reading for all women. It is a wonderful reminder of the importance of our girlfriends.

> **Maryanne Gale,** Vice President, Product Supply Asia, Procter & Gamble

Friendships provide solace, energize our lives, and expand our opportunities for enjoyment of life. This book explains why. It will make you cherish the friends you have, re-establish friendships lost, and, perhaps, place an immediate call to catch up with an old friend.

> **Jean K. Cleary, Esq.,** Managing Attorney, New York State Department of Public Service

Magic is in sending the message of friendship to the ones we love!

> **Merri Gaither Smith,** Community leader

This is a MUST read! The authors speak directly from their hearts and through their experiences. That they have written such a lovely, insightful book clearly indicates that they share a profound friendship built from many pleasurable—and amusing—events, resolved challenges, and loyalty. They inspired me to look closely at my girlfriends, to rejoice in their diversity and be grateful for how much they have enriched my life.

> **Judith Harmony,** Director, Harmony Project

Women find it easy to share intimacies—to lend support, comfort, and empathy while celebrating each other's triumph and joy. This book honors these important relationships.

> **Charlene Ventura**, President and CEO, YWCA of Greater Cincinnati

This book is a wonderful reminder to all women to nurture their women friendships. It is easy to get caught up in busy lives, and forget to take time out with women friends. When you face a difficult situation, you can always count on your women friends to really listen and help and be there for you.

> **Francie Pepper**, Community leader

Life Begins and Ends with

GIRLFRIENDS

Judith Van Ginkel and Betsy Kyte Newman

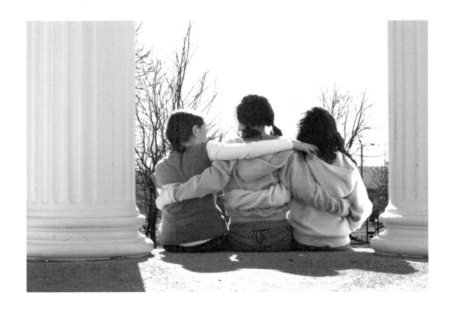

Cincinnati Book Publishers

Life Begins and Ends with Girlfriends

AUTHORS
Judith Van Ginkel
Betsy Kyte Newman

MANAGING EDITOR
Sue Ann Painter

PRODUCTION
Anthony W. Brunsman II

EDITOR
Mark P. Painter

COVER DESIGN
Brent Beck

TEXT DESIGN
Mark P. Painter

PHOTOGRAPHS
Helen Adams

Printed in the United States of America by
The John S. Swift Co. Inc.
First Edition, 2007
Published by Cincinnati Book Publishers
http:// www.cincybooks.com
ISBN: 0-9772720-7-9; 978-0-9772720-7-5

The book is available at a quantity discount for use in corporate training programs and for resale by nonprofit organizations as an educational and fundraising tool. See final pages of this book for order information.

Acknowledgments

Betsy and Judy
Cincinnati
2007

First, our profound thanks to all of you—the women and girls—who shared your stories and insights with us.

Our gratitude to our friends, who have taught us so much, and supported us through good times and sad times.

We are especially thankful for our beloved husbands, children, and (in Judy's case) grandchildren, who believe in us and have shown us the joy happy relationships can bring.

To the first readers and critics of the manuscript—our deep appreciation for your reviews.

To Sue Ann Painter and Tony Brunsman for their faith in—and encouragement for—the book project, thank you.

To Angie Coyle for her constant, cheerful support, incredible competence, and enthusiasm. There would be no book without you, Angie.

Life Begins and Ends with Girlfriends

Contents

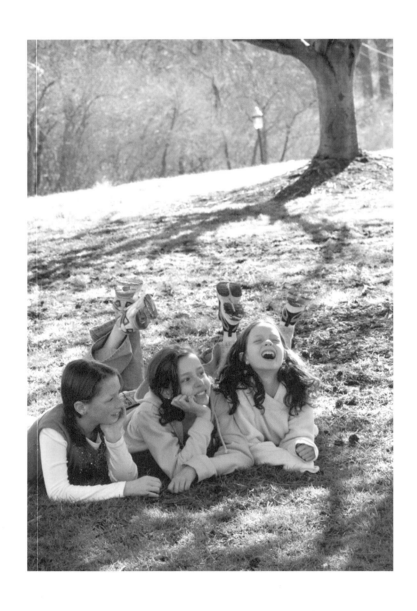

Why we wrote this book

Betsy Newman

Perhaps the story of our own friendship would be illuminating. We met in the fall of 1989 as new participants in Leadership Cincinnati, a program to train community volunteers to be more effective. Although we come from different backgrounds (Judy via West Virginia and Colorado, Betsy a product of Cincinnati who has lived in San Francisco and Boston), our friend chemistry was instant and mutual. We saw things the same way, we were similarly dedicated to balancing family and work, both at midlife, and—most importantly—we laughed at the same things!

In fact, laughter was our shared and favorite form of communication through that whole fascinating and intense year. Following Leadership Cincinnati, we stayed in touch and our friendship flourished over lunches, talks, coffees, community projects, and frivolous girl-talk for 17 years. When Judy mentioned that she'd wanted to write a book on friendship, I confessed that that was my own secret hope and—voila! We decided to collaborate. As a bonus, our shared writing project (undertaken with some fear as to how it might damage a precious friendship) has only enhanced our friendship. Because of our working together, we feel closer than ever! Thinking about friendship has made our own friendship even more priceless.

Let us answer a few questions at the start. Do we think we are experts on friendship? Only to the extent that we have not only reflected on our own experiences over two lifetimes, but have also had the benefit of listening to and reading the comments of the women and girls we surveyed in our research. Their accumulated wisdom, along with our own, is the heart of this book.

Secondly, why don't we deal in our book with male-female friendship? We simply feel that fascinating but complex subject goes beyond the territory of this book, which is the "simple" but profound landscape of women's friendships.

And finally, why this book now? Because we think female friendships are different now because our lives are different from those of our foremothers. We may have less time, more mobility, and fewer lifelong friends than did our mothers and grandmothers, but never has friendship, we feel, been more necessary to our mental and physical health. In short, a consideration and celebration of girlfriendships seemed eminently timely.

Judy Van Ginkel

You are probably asking yourself: "Who are these women and why do they think that they have something to teach me about friendship? Friendship is easy. I have friends. You have friends. Why in the world would anyone need lessons in friendship?" Our answer to you is this: We live in chaotic times, typically away from relatives and people who have known us since childhood. Our lives are busy. We have lost the safety net that sustained our mothers and grandmothers. We have misplaced the markers that gave direction to our lives—even when we didn't want them, didn't think we needed them.

We find ourselves reaching for human connection and the people who most often touch us are friends—neighbor friends, work friends, gym-and-club friends, parents-of-children friends. As you will note as you read through our book, friends move through our lives—some staying for many years and others for a shorter visit. You find these friends serving as sisters, aunts, mothers, or daughters, but without the familial bonds that can provide solace and security and be constricting at the same time.

It is important to us and we hope, important to you, that you think carefully and deeply about who your friends are and how you relate to them. Our book, *Life Begins and Ends with Girlfriends,* is written to help you begin that thinking process. In some cases, we offer permission: "celebrate the temporary, don't be afraid to say goodbye, take chances, be real." In other places, we provide advice: girlfriendships can teach you how to handle failure; be brave enough to bring strong feelings into your life; a girlfriendship bank can sustain you over a lifetime; it is the *friend* part that matters, not the *best* part.

We have found as we have talked with more than 100 girls and women that it is oh-so-important to take the time to reflect about your girlfriendships—friends from years ago and friends from today. We all choose to remember those people and situations that have been important to us. As you reminisce, the fabric of your life will begin to emerge. One thought will lead to another, and you will begin to extract—perhaps more consciously than you ever have before—lessons and patterns. We have. The women who talked with us and completed our questionnaires have. We have found ourselves making lists of stories we wanted to remember and even of some we would rather forget. You will find yourself seeing your constellation of friends in an entirely new way and perhaps, as we have, embracing the understanding of what friendship has meant in your life.

We promise that if you take our advice and spend time thinking in a focused way about your girlfriendships—who they have been, what they have meant, how the relationships were sustained or ended, what you have learned—your life will be enriched, and you will find yourself valuing your girlfriends and embracing them in a different but perhaps more accepting way.

There are lessons here for women of our age and for women considerably younger. The issues may be different; the landscape changed, but know that your girlfriends will sustain you. Treasure them. We begin life with girls—our mothers, our sisters, our friends and at the end of life, the faces may be different but our girls are still there. Life begins and ends with girlfriends. How fortunate we are to have each other.

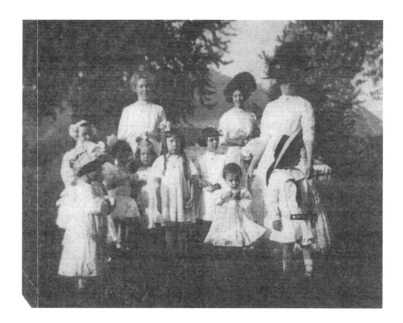

Introduction

Dear Reader:

We have often remarked that the unique and powerful bond of girlfriendship sustains us over our life span. For a woman, we believe, life begins and ends with her girlfriends. As we have talked with friends, professional colleagues, and women of different ages, we have been struck not only by their agreement with this statement but also their willingness to talk about it. They have been eager to help us create a commentary on girlfriendships and to become part of an accumulated wisdom about women's friendships that we could send to our sisters.

We interviewed nearly 100 girls and women, ages 10–98, and have woven their thinking with our own beliefs about friendship, sometimes using their actual words, and sometimes paraphrasing. We present their thoughts here with our commentary. Because we value friendships so much, we knew our findings were a legacy we wanted to leave, and so we share them with you.

Please read this book over our shoulders—read as if you were having a conversation with a trusted friend. A book, we know, doesn't replace a dialogue between two people but it is there for you to hold in your hand, to go back to, to comment on, to mark up with your own ideas and observations.

In short, this book that began as ours, we want to be truly yours. This book, with your own notes and memories, can be a source of solace; it can offer explanation or validation. It can prompt you to just spend a few minutes thinking freely about girlfriends from your past and your present. Who comes into your mind? Why? What do you remember? In all cases, our memories have an edit function. What occurs to you is there for a reason—tangible expressions of joy or healing or outrage. We promise that you will find this small exercise insightful and stimulating. This book can be your own private journal or you can use it to leave reflections and explanations for others. How many of you have wanted to know more long after someone important to you has gone—a mother, an aunt, a sister, a daughter, a friend? What mattered to them? What hurt? What brought gladness? What lessons would they like to impart if they could right now?

You, our readers, can do that for those you love and, in the process, illuminate your life for yourself. This intimate experience provides a way to say what you may not be able to articulate.

So here goes. We hope that these thoughts will cause you to reflect about signal girlfriendship events in your own life—the people, the times, the experiences. For us, our writing has provided a stimulus to introspection; it has caused us to remember and reflect about our girlfriends over many decades. We hope that you will have that experience. You will find that as you begin to focus on what female companionship and close friendship has meant to you, the richness of these memories will astonish you. You will come to understand that your girlfriendships have been—and continue to be—incredibly important and life affirming, even though they involve risks and challenges, may not last forever, and sometimes disappoint you.

Girlfriend relationships also have the power to be magically rewarding: they often result in long-term mental and physical benefits. Studies consistently prove that well-being and health are enhanced by having friends. Apparently, all of us function better when we have strong social bonds. Our friends keep us centered and connected. When life gets tough and we'd like to give up; our friends can be there, surrounding us with love and encouragement. They can help us to hang on when we are not sure that is possible. For this and more, friendship is worth the efforts and risks involved. Remember though, that it is a Hallmark illusion to believe that all friendships are cherished, nurtured, and nurturing. We all know that the rewards of friendship can be accompanied by loss and betrayal.

Women change—relationships change, for all kinds of reasons or no apparent reason at all. Not all friendships are true and life-enhancing. We hope to provide you with the resources to handle loss and the courage to try again—we believe that friendships are worth the time and effort.

Our friends help to define us at all stages of life, but most dramatically at its beginning and end. At the dawn of life, friends help shape us, and at life's sunset, they provide us support and a kind of reference point on the meaning of our lives. So much of who we are results from our girlfriendships and the influences they exert.

Please join us on this journey in celebration of women's friendships. We hope you will find, as we have, that your circle of friends becomes a family circle for you—present, understanding, and supporting. We hope that the ideas expressed here provide validation for you and for your girlfriendships. This book is meant to be a guide along the pathway to true and life-affirming relationships.

Sincerely,

Judy and Betsy

Women care for each other and each other's families. We dry each other's tears and cheer each other on. We carry each other until we are strong enough to walk alone. In short, women create a caring community— friendship is woman's special province.

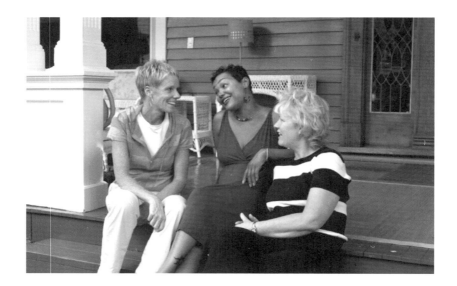

CHAPTER 1

Celebrating Girlfriendships

Let us celebrate girlfriendships—those essential strands that are woven into the fabric of a woman's life. Girlfriendships, which provide women with strong and sustaining bonds, have rarely been given their full due of respect and honor. We hope to remedy this slight.

What has always struck us about girlfriendships is this: they are a connection that, even though often relegated to the sidelines, can be steadfastly there for nourishment and support.

For most of us, the unspoken truth is this: our plans with girlfriends are often subject to change according to the needs of our family. What we want you—our readers and our own daughters and granddaughters—to notice is that life *begins* and *ends* with our girlfriends. Girlfriends are there at the very beginning of girlhood to help define and grow us and, at the end of life, when so many other relationships have faded or disappeared. They remain as our witness and support, giving testimony to the lives we have led. In celebrating girlfriendships, we hope to encourage your own realization of the lifelong value of your girlfriendships.

How girlfriend relationships are different

Girlfriendships are different from other relationships in your lives and should not be confused with acquaintanceships—though those are part of life too. Your girlfriends shape your lives and even define you as people. The old adage, "Show me who your friends are and I will tell you who you are" is true. Friendship is a confirmation of the self; your choice of friends explains not only who you are, but also who you aspire to be.

Friendship is founded on an interesting dynamic because, while you choose your friends, they choose you too. You may remember making unfortunate (or even disastrous) girlfriendship choices in adolescence when cliques and the lust for popularity ruled your decisions.

Betsy writes:

I remember being in junior high school and yearning to be in the "cool" group in my all-girls school. I tried for a long time to imitate and cultivate Anne and Peggy, the quintessential blondes, with their smooth pageboys and lazy smiles–even though I was much too bookish, dorky, and shy to ever be considered remotely "cool." They were not unkind, and tried to be gracious and inclusive, but it became obvious after a few weeks that I was a poor fit into their clique, and I was gradually dropped. I simply was no longer invited to join them.

I remember the day of my final disgrace vividly. It happened at lunchtime—that time of sharpest distinction—when those who were popular sat together, easily enjoying the privilege of the elite, the chosen. I had been in the habit of sitting at Anne and Peggy's table, where they had kindly, if absently, tolerated me. Amid the clank of dishes and trays, I proceeded as usual to their table to be greeted with awkward silence and lowered eyes. "Oh, hi . . .." Anne said weakly. "I'm sorry . . . uh . . . we're saving that seat for somebody else." As if it were today, I remember the weight of my tray and my hot flush of shame as I stumbled to the next empty table and sat alone. A classic, almost cliché-like tale of junior-high rejection and angst. And yet so much more. That was the beginning of self-knowledge for me.

Of course, I was devastated, but recovered and found my place and footing with three precious friends who became my true soul mates throughout high school. Nancy, Patty, and Cathy helped me define myself and navigate the shoals of growing up, and I remain both close and grateful to them today.

In those critical "growing up" years, when you begin to look beyond your birth family to shape yourself, your peer group and your chosen friends act as a kind of yardstick to help you measure yourself. During the teen years, your friends seem to hold your very selves and your budding identities in their hands. Just when your family begins to view you and your new independence with alarm and some distaste, your friends are there to help nurture your new identity.

You can find true friends in any age group. You will have older as well as younger soul mates—elder mentor-friends to teach you and validate you, and younger learning-friends for when you are the touchstone.

Distinguishing true friends from false friends

How can one distinguish true friendship from the many and good acquaintanceships that enhance women's lives?

First, your girlfriends are, in a sense, soul mates with whom you experience a meeting of hearts as well as minds. One woman describes friendship as an "almost psychic bond of recognition." What we hope you recognize in your friends is a level of trustworthiness and mutual respect that provides fertile ground for growing friendship. You need to be sure that your friends are worthy to share your deepest secrets and will guard them safely. Time, trust, and basic sharing of values are necessary to grow such bonds. Our survey respondents agreed that the emblem of authentic friendship is the ease with which they could disclose personal feelings, faults, and issues.

Friends will allow you to be your own true self. With your good and trusted friends, you won't feel the pressure to be "entertaining," to put on a happy face, or wear a false front. As Judy's father used to say, "Friends don't need explanations; enemies won't believe them." (Funny how often these old sayings prove to be true!)

True friends are there when you need them

Keep in mind that it is often when you are in trouble that, as you have heard so many times before, you find out who your friends are. You will be surprised that the people who reach out to you are often not those you would expect.

Judy's divorce provides a graphic story. Other women saw her as either a threat or a promise—a threat because they were afraid that she wanted their husbands or a promise because they were in bad marriages and unsure what to do about them. At first, married couples took her out and included her in parties and trips to see the children at summer camp. She was euphoric for about a year, lauding herself for finally having the courage to face her demons.

Often, she accepted their invitations while becoming increasingly uncomfortable with them. (Who picks up the dinner check? Am I talking with the male person too long and not including the woman? Am I intruding? Did they invite me out of obligation or genuine interest in spending time together?) You get the gist. The couple's invitations began to taper off and Judy began to refuse them when they came. Rather, she spent time with women—mostly single women—who had interests similar to her own. Sometimes these women were also divorcees and in a few cases they were still married but willing to be engaged beyond their couples world.

Be sure to keep in mind when selecting friends that your own feelings are impeccable. You know when you look forward to seeing someone or when you feel comfortable calling with a problem. And, you have all experienced the hurt that comes when you ask a girlfriend to help and she finds an excuse—and then begins to distance herself from you. You may think to yourself that this woman is not worthy of your friendship. But before you dismiss her entirely, try to find out what happened and whether there were difficulties in her life that left little energy for anyone else at the time.

Woman's special province

It is in our tendency to befriend, to embrace, to bond, and to gather together that our woman's gift becomes most clear. Women care for each other and each other's families; we dry each other's tears and cheer each other on. We carry each other until we are strong enough to walk alone. In short, women create a caring community. Although some men may dispute this, we hope that you share our belief that friendship is woman's special province.

We may select our friends

One of the prerequisites of friendship we want you to discover is an understanding about yourself and your own needs. While friendship is often initially motivated by self-interest, it is perpetuated through mutual interest. Your own psychological and emotional barriers affect your willingness to search for and even to accept friendship.

Most girls and women say that they want to have girlfriends but some women are hard to be friends with. Or maybe they will be your good and true friends for a while—and then their situation and yours will change. You suddenly (or not so suddenly) realize that the shared core values and interests that held you together are no longer there. And keep in mind that good friendships may not last forever.

Judy explains to her daughters:

Let me give you an example that goes back to the time when you were small. I became friendly with a woman I met soon after I moved to Cincinnati. This woman and I exchanged parties. You played with her children. We had lunch and gossiped about what was going on in town. But gradually I began to realize that our conversations were primarily about her and her problems, which, I must admit, were real. She had a sick child. She was ill herself. Her marriage gave her little comfort. Yet, she had many resources, a keen and inquiring mind, and access to help. I began to understand that I was only part of her larger support system— one more person in a long line of counselors and doctors. The difference was that they were paid to be interested. I was looking for a friend who could listen to me, and I was more than willing to listen to her. But there needs to be mutuality for the relationship to continue.

The relationship dissolved when I told her about my recent separation from my husband, and I described what my life had been like for the past months—acrimony, fear, threats, taunting, and derisive words. She listened for a while, then told me that what I really needed to do to feel better was to redo my kitchen. The kitchen was outdated, she said, and the remodeling process would surely make me feel better. I thanked her for her suggestion. I paid the lunch check and left.

About the same time, another girl I thought of as a friend called to chat. She told me that she had just had the worst day of her life. Of course, I asked what happened. Well, she said, they discontinued the fabric that she had selected for her living room. My day had begun and ended with an ex-husband who came into my house, sorted through the mail, went into the refrigerator, began eating our dinner, and then threatened to take my children away. There was no way at that time in my life that I could be comforted with superficialities. I found myself searching for new friends who could live life at a different level. And the strange thing was that these new friends did not share history with me as did the two women in the stories above. Yet, these new girlfriends would talk with me for hours about their lives and mine. They were less involved with life's material things; they read poetry and philosophy books; they went to foreign films and saw astrologists; and they were fun. Younger than I, without children, but willing and able to warm to someone new and provide comfort in the dead of winter.

Girlfriendships are created by many bonds

Sometimes friendships that begin with self-interest can grow into relationships with more depth when you can find mutual interest.

Judy remembers:

A year ago an old friend died. A friend of long standing—more than forty years. She was a woman who lived many years—just over 100. Words to describe her: irascible, clever, smart, funny, and the best antique dealer I will ever know. We met one another when I signed up for her antique class soon after moving to Cincinnati. Hattie helped me decorate two houses and, along the way, we spent part of most Saturdays together. We went all over southern Ohio and northern Kentucky looking for early things that met her standards and my taste. And were we successful!

I came to know her well and understand her childhood, the early death of her husband, the life of a woman alone in the business world when women were staying home and tending to family. She was considerably older than I, but we learned from one another and formed a friendship that I miss even today. Often when I am planning my Saturdays, I think about Hattie and the fun we had together. We were never social friends and other than a party or two, we limited our time together to Saturday outings. But those Saturdays and our mutual interest in 17th and 18th century furniture and things "of the period" allowed us to develop a friendship from a business relationship.

Our lives are replete with situations that encourage two people to get together for self-interest. It isn't necessarily bad and often it is practical—the person you study with, the one who shares the car pool, the girl who likes to travel with you or play tennis. These relationships work and are basic to us as we move through our days and weeks. But occasionally in these settings, we find someone with whom we resonate, and we find ourselves seeking this person outside of the bounds of the expected encounters. We think of it as mutuality of interest rather than just mutual interest. And for us that denotes establishing bonds of trust, and candor, and kindness.

An example here. Judy speaks of a woman she has worked with for almost ten years: "She is younger than I, grew up in a large family of girls, and is simply one of the nicest people I know. We came together to work, but as the months passed, we also became friends. She asks about problems, knows what I am worried about, is never judgmental, and is always trustworthy. We laugh together and overlay humor on the most bizarre experiences. The feelings that I describe I know are mutual. Our relationship gives color and richness to our lives; we have fun, and we value one another. That defines girlfriendship, doesn't it?"

Perhaps the most important truth we can reveal to you is that girlfriendships are created by many bonds that are woven together to form a mantle of love and protection. Girlfriendships are not right or wrong. Girlfriendship means experiencing life's joy and adversity together with the understanding that even your girlfriends will not, cannot, always be there. Much of life you will experience alone.

Consider the widow who told us that her aloneness was terrifying to some of her girlfriends. They just wanted her to be "all right" after her husband died so that they could relieve their own anxiety. With them, this widow pretended. On the surface, she was strong and calm, which made it easier for her girlfriends. Then, she went home to cry alone. She quickly identified the girlfriends who could see her pain and hold her feelings; these were—and are—the girlfriends who moved forward with her.

For us and for most of the women we call girlfriends, truthfulness and trust are essential to a girlfriendship. Can you be who you are pretending to be someone else? How candid are you willing to be? How candid can you be? How much honesty can you tolerate? Will you allow yourself to be vulnerable? We have lived too long and seen too much to be willing to tolerate platitudes, socially acceptable answers, and untrustworthy behavior. You need honest responses to your questions and someone to tell you what you might not want to hear—but need to hear. You have legions of acquaintances, but as you become more insightful about yourself and closer to your feelings, your expectations for your girlfriendships will be higher. One woman in her 60s, when asked if she ever maintained "superficial" or shallow friendships told us, "I suppose I do, but I don't really enjoy these as much and am increasingly spending less time with people with whom I can't be real."

Indeed, paradoxically, it is in times of your greatest need that you will discover the strength of your friendship bonds. One cancer survivor told us, "So many good friends have literally held me and supported me through this whole ordeal. I have never felt so loved. This fearful time gave me a chance to demonstrate love, which is too often unspoken." All of us remember who dried our tears, who helped us. Our friends chant a mantra that becomes a chorus (in which we concur) when they say that the older we get the more important are our female friendships.

In the end we all learn that it is relationships—girlfriendships—that matter.

Ideas to think about

- Friends help shape our lives, define us as people, and reveal our true selves.
- Celebrate your girlfriendships.
- One of the prerequisites of friendship is understanding yourself.

My thoughts

-
-
-

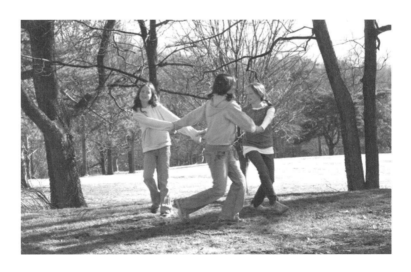

When you can acknowledge your failures and weaknesses along with your triumphs, then and only then, do you have the basis for a strong and enduring girlfriendship.

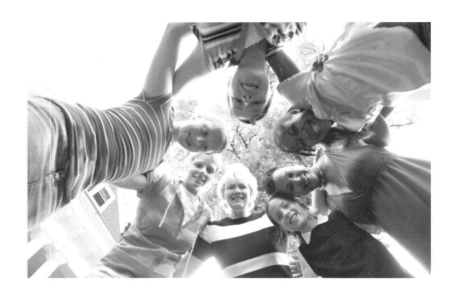

CHAPTER 2

Friendships Change over Time

Modern American women's lives typically begin and end with girlfriends. But between the beginning and the ending are the years, the months, the days, the hours that comprise our lives. How are our girlfriendships woven into that fabric and are these relationships different now than they were even 20 or 30 years ago? When we asked these questions of our survey group of women and girls, we received remarkably consistent responses.

Certainly, the environment has changed over the past 30 years: more women work, more women divorce, more women live away from their family homes and relatives. We are healthier, live longer, and retire earlier. We live in a world that is increasingly more fragmented and mobile. These trends have been accelerating and have led, we believe, to new roles and different expectations for women.

To young women, girlfriendships are primary. Young women need friends to do things with. They need to test their social skills and their perceptions of the world. They find safety in numbers and yearn for a best friend, a group of friends, a clique. Together they learn. Each of us has had those experiences. We have experienced the joy that comes with belonging and the sadness that comes when the best friend drops us, or the girlfriend group breaks apart, or the group leaves us out, inflicting the suffering of a poignant—and devastating—loss.

As males enter the constellation, dynamics change again, and often relationships with girlfriends become secondary to those with the boyfriend, the male friend, the husband. Put yourself in this picture and fast forward . . . college, career, young married, children. Girlfriends can still be there and you can still find solace, comfort, happiness, and humor with them. But too often your time with them is limited. You just simply don't have the energy to nurture a girlfriendship.

Keep moving forward: children are grown, your immediate life needs are met, you may or may not have a male partner. You look around and, if you are very lucky (and maybe smart), there are girlfriends—old friends from childhood, new friends from work, or clubs, or the neighborhood. In mid-career, or midlife, or both, you will find yourself beginning to enjoy and benefit from strong friendships with women based on mutual respect and a shared sense—as one woman put it—of the "ridiculous nature of life."

Time and experience are on our side

As we age, we develop more self-confidence about our girlfriendships. We have rejoiced in some and suffered through others. We know what we can tolerate and what brings us pleasure. We have a more attenuated sense of which personalities mesh best with our own. And maybe our ego needs are minimized, and we can enter into a more satisfying, more real, girlfriendship.

As we all move between our own reality and the worlds of our mothers and grandmothers, keep in mind that women now in their late 50s and 60s are part of the first generation of girls who left home for college and did not come back. Often, our adult girlfriendships grow outside of our hometown rather than with childhood friends. Our options for friendships are broader than those that were available to our mothers and grandmothers. Gradually, we have developed wisdom about relationships as our mothers and grandmothers did, but this learning has occurred in a milieu—an environment—that is dramatically different.

Many women told us that they asked themselves whether the differences between their girlfriendships and those of their mothers and grandmothers were due to a change in the ways we are able to communicate now, or whether they were a function of the time available, or the expected role of a woman in a family. Historically, husband and children always came first and the psychosocial needs of the woman, the mother, were the last to be addressed. Women had fewer opportunities to meet other women outside of their own social class or family-interest groups. They were not expected even to have girlfriendships on their own, much less discuss their problems, their hopes, and desires with a non-family member.

Most of the women we interviewed did not think that their mothers and grandmothers had girlfriendships that were as intimate as those today. Why? In years past, there was a stronger focus on taking care of home, husband, and children. That is what a woman, a mother, a wife was supposed to do. She was confined to a domestic sphere. In the late twentieth century, she slowly came out into the larger world. Several women used the word "sacrifice" to describe the traditional and historic role of women.

Judy writes to her daughters:

Your grandmother was 98 when she explained to me that her family members have been her friends and she hasn't needed other people to help solve her problems. She said that she has rarely discussed family issues with anyone outside of the family and that her family relationships have filled her need for girlfriendships. However, her husband (your grandfather) died 18 years ago at age 80. Mother needed to find companionship with neighbors and childhood friends. Her last girlfriend died three years ago on the anniversary of granddaddy's death. Today, she talks about loneliness and isolation. Her husband gone, the women she thought of as girlfriends dead, her children out of town, and with the seclusion made possible with economic security, she is alone at the most melancholy and frightening time of her life.

Your grandmother found younger friends with mutual interests. They go to movies, out to dinner, and to an occasional play, but these women do not share her history and the voice that was spoken through most of her life is silent. She tells stories from the past over and then over again. She wants to remember the grand trip to Europe, traveling through Germany in 1938, moving into the house where she lives now, her brother's visits and getting dressed up for lunch. We—the daughters—listen, but even we are a generation apart. We didn't know her as a young girl when she met my father, when she graduated from high school, when her mother, my elegant grandmother, died.

Betsy remembers:

My own mother remains a poignant example of the power of friendship even (and especially) at the end of her long life. At the age of 98, she had outlived most of her girlhood pals and women friends, yet those who remained were deeply cherished. She loved her monthly sewing group (most members were decades younger, but enjoyed her company) and her French club, that endured from 1928 until the membership dwindled 70 years later. She adored talking with old and new friends and relished making new friends, especially younger ones.

She taught me the value of adding new friends as life goes on, and of living in the present and remaining engaged with life through younger friends. Incredibly, she continued to attend her beloved college reunions from 1928 through 2003, her 75th! What an example she is to us of the enduring power—and sustaining bond—of friendship.

Wisdom handed down the generations

Our children all have had the joy of having grandmothers know them as adults. They have heard about their lives as girls and been able to ask questions of their elders nearing the end of their lives. The children watched as their grandmothers deteriorated and friends died. They have seen what aloneness can do and how important companionship is. Their grandmothers outlived friends and husbands. They told the younger generations what has truly mattered in their lives: family and girlfriends.

Women's opportunities for friendship have grown

It is possible to make good and firm girlfriendships in later life— friendships not based on a long history but more often on mutual need. These girlfriendships have value in themselves and for the time they exist, but because they cannot have the richness of a girlfriendship that spans the years, they are more similar to annual flowers than a perennial garden. Like annuals, they are brilliant, vibrant, and short-lived. Perennials have less color, but they offer steady, dependable growth.

It appears that the differences between our girlfriendships and those of our mothers and grandmothers are not differences of loyalty or trust, but rather changes in the ways we are able to reach out for girlfriendships with people who have diverse views and interests—girls and women who may or may not be from the same cultural environment. And then, having entered into girlfriendships, we are more willing to discuss personal issues and to share feelings, including strong, or embarrassing, or revealing thoughts. Our mothers and grandmothers carried their individual burdens by themselves, not wanting to appear weak or emotional, even with good friends. It just "wasn't done" and was seen as betrayal of husband and family. The circles were small and the options for candor limited.

Today, women have opportunities to develop girlfriendships with new and different people and to have a broader social outlook. One young woman characterized it this way—she felt that both her mother and her grandmother were "forced" into relationships with wives of their husband's friends and associates, but that she has more choices and more freedom. She doesn't see geographic separation as a barrier because she can use email, voicemail, and instant messaging to maintain frequent and close contact with distant girlfriends. In years past, it was either writing letters (a dead art?) or talking on the telephone. Judy remembers vividly the days when the long distance telephone bill would come to her house and her father would complain that it was close to the national debt. Well, today you can talk all day for pennies. You can talk while you are on a walk, shopping, driving, even wandering through a museum. Be clear, we are not advocating relationship-by-voice-mail, but we surely need to acknowledge that it is easier to be in contact with someone today than it was in years past. It is the absence of content not the contact that is suspect.

Although we can technically communicate with friends and family, in an important way, we are more isolated and alone than ever before. We are often amazed when we are with a group of women and no one is talking with the person in front of or beside them. Rather, these women are having inane, almost frantic, conversations on their cell phones. Later one of them may say, "It was nice spending time with you," when, in truth, you were just there trying to carry on what became a disjointed conversation between phone calls. One or two experiences like that, and we guess that you are busy the next time that woman calls to make plans.

Electronics—cell phones, email, instant messaging—all promote communication that is impersonal, indifferent, and distracting. Or, even worse, these devices are used to send a disturbing message when facing the person would be too painful. Think back. Hasn't that happened to you? How often have you received an important email message embedded with other emails that are routine junk mail? If only our security service could protect us from hurtful people and the sadness they inflict.

Allow friendships to happen

But girlfriendship isn't simply talking with another woman. Rather, it is your willingness to be honest and vulnerable, to allow the girlfriendship to become real. You can construct a façade of perfection that stands for a while, but something always happens that allows you to know that you are neither perfect nor impervious. As parents, often those events occur when your children become adolescents, or as a wife when your marriage breaks up, or your parents die, or your friends become ill.

Betsy recalls:

I can pinpoint the day when my regular, if casual, lunches with Patti and Rita changed from exchanging friendly chitchat to close friendship: it was the moment when I let down my guard. Driven by the sheer need to communicate, I shared my parental worries. My perfect son was going through a rebellious period and was causing us much worry and tension. I was ashamed to confess my shortcomings as a mother, but they saw the tears I tried to brush away as I haltingly told my story. "I don't know what to do," I managed finally. "Oh, Betsy, it's all right . . . we know . . . we've been there. It happens . . . hang in and you'll be all right." Patti and Rita figuratively and literally embraced me with understanding, compassion, and the benefit of their own considerable parenting expertise.

When I dropped the mask of perfection and competence and revealed my own truth, a real friendship emerged and flourished. With relief, I learned I didn't have to pretend to be perfect and all together to be loved and accepted by true friends.

Some assembly required

Required: your willingness to be open, and a trusted friend willing to listen. When you can acknowledge your failures and weaknesses along with your triumphs, then and only then, do you have the basis for a strong and enduring girlfriendship. This opportunity is available to you if you are willing and able to take the risks to make it happen. For our mothers and grandmothers, that choice was largely absent.

We believe that younger women see their girlfriendships as more permanent than do older women who have had more life experience and probably more disappointment. The young girls believe that their girlfriendships from school, neighborhoods, clubs, and camp will continue forever and that nothing, nothing is more important. Older women better understand impermanence. They treasure history and continuity, but they are not fogged by illusion. Knowing even temporary relationships are meaningful, as women age, they turn to girlfriends—old and new. They may resurrect old friendships or search for brand-new friendships, but the specter of aloneness propels these women to seek out companions, playmates, and counselors.

Ending a friendship

Sometimes it is kinder to end a girlfriendship than to continue to foster hope in another person or, for that matter, in yourself. Apply the pleasure-pain principle and calibrate whether the pain outweighs the pleasure. You will know—each of us is an expert in recognizing how we feel. Trust your instincts, and understand that separating allows both of you to look elsewhere for more satisfying girlfriendships. Don't feel guilty. If you find a girlfriend constantly draining, then maybe she isn't a good match for you. Keep in mind that if parting is well made, you may be able to gather together again. So we say, maybe there is "nothing there but the history," but the history has created who we are.

One woman said that when she was younger she was more willing to get close to others more quickly and then later had

31

regrets. She explained that, as she grew older, she had fewer girlfriendships but the ones she did have were deeper and more intimate. She credits her ability to be more honest with herself and more selective about whom she allows into her "inner self." She has formed more limited, but more satisfying late relationships.

Family relationships prepare us for friendships

Love and friendship within a family prepare us for loving friendships outside—and make the assumption that there are good and fine relationships that do not end. Death, geographic distance, life changes lead to relationship changes. But a good connection between two people transcends these barriers, preparing us for other successful and enduring friendships.

Judy says that although her father died 18 years ago, he is still with her. Because he believed in her, he is not gone from her. She can feel him standing by her as she works her way through her life. She examines problems and situations and knows what he would say about them. And, of course, there are times when she has tears in her eyes—he is not here to see his great-grandchildren, it is Father's Day, she just visited a place with outstanding fly-fishing streams and he would have reveled in being there.

Losing her father was incredibly difficult, but she has never been sorry that her feelings were strong or that she was devastated when he died. He taught her that last final lesson when he told her as he was dying that his life was extraordinary and that he wouldn't have wanted to miss one minute—the good and the bad. Isn't that what each and every one of us want from a friendship? And don't these people, the ones who influenced our lives, stay with us forever?

Ideas to think about

- Remember that as you grow older you will need your girlfriends even more than you think you do now.
- You have the opportunity now to look broadly to find a girlfriend or girlfriends with whom you can share trust and candor.
- Sometimes it is kinder to end a girlfriendship than to continue when the connection is broken.
- Allow yourself to be real; allow true friendships to happen.
- Even "lost" relationships stay with us and become part of who we are.

My thoughts

-
-
-

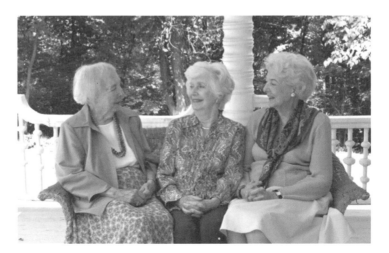

You take risks and may receive joy or sadness in return. But choose to live with passion and gusto, courage not fear.

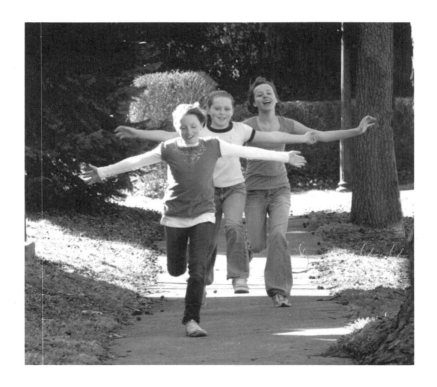

CHAPTER 3

Choose to Live with Passion

An individual's willingness to risk being a girlfriend is directly related to how she feels about herself. Exposing your feelings to others is often uncomfortable. You may not be sure that you want someone else to know about your weaknesses, your hopes, your disappointments. You are probably afraid that if someone knows you are soft, she will take advantage of you. You are aware that it hurts more to have and to lose than to have not risked your feelings in the first place. But we hope you also realize that to have great girlfriendships you have to be willing to expose even your most vulnerable side.

We want you to know that girlfriendship has great rewards and is well worth the risks. Have enough confidence in yourself to believe that, should the relationship falter, you can learn from it, grow above it, and go on. Choose wisely, of course. Look for people who seem to be true to your values, who let you know that you are worthy. And then tread carefully, developing trust little by little.

Put away your fears

Be willing to try out a friendship. Just beginning doesn't mean you are committed for always and forever. Girlfriendships end for a variety of reasons: you grow in different directions geographically or emotionally, your needs change, you have an argument. Think of it as you would of dating a guy. If you were only willing to date the person with whom you might have a long-term relationship, you would miss many interesting, exciting, and rewarding experiences. Think back to what you have learned from each girlfriendship you have had. The variety, the complexity, and the joy will amaze you. Not all experiences are good, but there is not one from which you cannot learn.

So what are you afraid of:
- Being rejected?
- Being betrayed?
- Being used?
- Being belittled?
- Being seen as less than perfect?
- Being intimidated by others you perceive as having more than you do—intelligence, money, position, power?
- Disappointing your friends?
- Not having enough time to nurture the friendship?
- Making a commitment that you don't think you can fulfill?
- Being involved with someone you see as too needy and not being able to meet those needs?

It is a formidable list, isn't it? But these fears are the underpinning for all of your relationships. As Judy's father told her, you want to find people who will love you with all of your faults or perceived shortcomings, and not in spite of them. In truth, these fears are why finding trusted girlfriends is so important. You need someone to go to when the world is black, or you need your confidence boosted, or you just need someone to say, "Hey, you are great!"

We all have had experiences that have caused us to be wary. You don't forget the time when you weren't invited to a party, included in a movie trip, betrayed by someone you trusted. And yet, we try again. A friend of ours who is in her 60s said it well, "Taking a risk to try-out a friendship is not terminal and therefore a good incentive for forming one."

Judy remembers:

I still feel the sting that came when I was 13 and some girls were whispering about me in the hall. The one person I thought was my friend was right in the middle of the group, and I knew they were talking about me. She showed me that I couldn't trust her, and I went home in tears. The slights were everything from leaving me out when a group of girls got together to play Clue on a Sunday afternoon to walking off and leaving me alone after school. To this day, when this girl's name comes into my mind, I relive every agonizing moment.

And if you think that the early wounds ever completely heal, just try going to a class reunion. I did once and will never go again. It only takes a few minutes for the years to disappear and for you—and the people you went to high school with—to respond just as they did decades ago. I always got good grades, but in those days girls were not supposed to talk about that. Rather, it was better to be a majorette or a cheerleader, have a steady boyfriend—preferably an athlete—be fun, and have a blond pageboy haircut. I went to college, and I grew up and developed self-confidence. So, when the high school reunion invitation came, I decided that I could attend, not realizing that I would be as invisible now as I was then. The final insult came when they announced the people who had been in the National Honor Society and forgot to mention me. I lost hours, days, and weeks of sleep worrying for four years of high school about whether these girls liked me and how I could be part of their group. I was just fortunate to be able to get away, but I left that reunion early and did not return the second night. Invitations to another gathering are coming in the mail now, and they go where they belong for me, into the wastebasket. Those girls were not and are not my friends. Having discussed my feelings with other girls and women, I know that my experience is not unique.

You may think that the petty "who is going to sit where" is left behind when you leave junior high school. Far too often that is not true. I was invited to a Sunday evening dinner party for girls only. Hosted by a widow friend of mine, she asked me to come to meet her other female friends, and I was pleased to be included. All went well until it was time for the buffet dinner. I prepared a plate of food and went to a table where there were unoccupied seats. I placed my plate on the table and was told rudely that the seat I had chosen was for someone else—I would need to find another place to eat. Obviously I left, my face burning and my mind thinking wicked thoughts. I can intellectualize about that woman's insecurities and childish behavior, but I can also tell you that, even today in my sixth decade—it hurts. I doubt that there is one who cannot think of similar experiences—everyone from the popular cheerleader and basketball star to the shy and retiring student to the seemingly ever-confident homecoming queen. We have these experiences early—and again later—and they mark what risks we are willing to take to develop a friendship.

Some women choose to walk alone

There are women who choose not to form close girlfriendships. These women describe themselves as loners, and say that they are willing to help others, but never will move the relationship to a more intimate level where two people begin to talk about their feelings. When asked, these women couldn't tell us whether they consciously or unconsciously avoided girlfriendships. When they seek out other women at all, they no doubt choose ones for whom more superficial relationships are acceptable.

In truth, we all make choices about our close friends. Judy recalls that once she rejected the offer for a friendship by telling a woman, "I am sure you are a nice person, but I just don't have time to have another person in my life." Judy remembered that: "The woman called repeatedly to schedule lunch, breakfast, or dinner, and each time I made excuses—legitimate, but excuses nonetheless. It was true that I was busy, but sometimes you will find that you simply do not have the energy to develop yet another girlfriendship." Declining an offer of close friendship may not be about your willingness to take a risk, but rather a reasonable and logical assessment about what you can accept into your life. We are here to tell you that is alright too.

Risks are relative

Risk, as we have explained, has many definitions. But our definition of risk always and forever must be forged against the experiences of one of our oldest respondents. At age 94, this warm, articulate, and intelligent woman talked of her years growing up as a young Jewish woman in Hungary during World War II. In that context, the risk of trusting the wrong person could be death.

Esther, a 94-year-old Holocaust survivor, remembers a chance meeting on the train taking her to the concentration camp in

Germany that led to the discovery of a lifelong and life-changing friendship. Here she describes meeting her first best friend en route to the concentration camp:

From the first moment we looked at each other, our conversation sounded like we could finish sentences together. She was my best friend, a super intelligent, always interesting, fine-behaving, decent, good human being. As long as life will be given to me, I will cherish her. What company! Two serious people meet under unusual circumstances. Why, for heaven's sake? In wartime, by accident, as war prisoners traveling together in cattle cars. Is this true, could this be happening?

Risk in the extreme. Yet, even in those circumstances, human connection provided the link to survival. How many of us could echo Ester's wonder and delight at discovering a kindred spirit in such dire circumstances!

Fortunately, most of us will not be tested in the way that this courageous woman was. But that is not to say that we won't be sad, and scared, and hurt. Just know that you learn from difficult experiences as well as from the more pleasant ones.

Judy recalls:

A personal experience brought this way of thinking home to me. I had a friend—a close and intimate friend—with whom I had weathered some difficult life experiences, including divorce, teenage children, angry and vengeful ex-husbands. We laughed together, we talked and processed our feelings, and we analyzed the issues. And late at night when everything just got too dark, we would talk on the phone until early into the morning. Having a sense of humor got us through so that we could go out and face each day. I believed that the relationship was working for both of us until one day I needed to call her. I tried for almost a week with no response—multiple phone calls, numerous messages. Finally, I got a note in the mail chiding me for being a pest and telling me that she would call when she was ready, not when I was. I didn't understand what happened then, and I don't understand now. She would never explain. Although later we did talk by phone a few times, she decided that for reasons she couldn't discuss, she couldn't be friends with me. It took me a long time to be able to venture into that kind of girlfriendship again, but eventually I did. The form of the girlfriendship was different because, by that time, I had remarried and my emotional and time commitments had changed. I still see this woman occasionally and although we greet one another warmly, now and forever I feel dropped, with my feelings splattered all over the ground and my confidence shattered.

But there is a lesson here. That lesson is that you go on and you do not, must not, judge all girlfriendships by one that has been hurtful. This woman and I were able to work our way through a thicket together, and there was great benefit in that experience alone. Together we learned gallows humor, and we laughed when the alternative was to cry. We found a way to get through each new day, and I think we both grew stronger. I mourn for the girlfriendship. I wish it were still possible to be together, but it isn't. So, I moved forward, treasuring what we had and being willing to embrace other girlfriendships again.

You will make your own decisions about girlfriendship. The point is to know that you have some control over your life. You take risks and may receive joy or sadness in return. But choose to live with passion and gusto, courage not fear. Always remember that no one can take away your memories and your experiences. At the end of life we are all alone and it is the remembered relationships of our life that sustain us. Work hard to have girlfriendships that warm you when the days are short and the air is thin.

Salvaging an endangered relationship

If you haven't already, one of these days you will find yourself at an impasse in a girlfriendship. Something has happened to cause the relationship to cool, you are uncomfortable together, and at least one of you is avoiding the other. What to do? First, you need to determine how important this girlfriendship is to you and whether you want to try to save it. A sister? An old friend? A friend in the midst of turmoil? Or someone you met in the women's club and joined for lunch or couples dinner on Saturday nights? For someone that you cherish, you may need to forget your pride and your ego and figure out how you can approach this person in the most positive way. A letter? A phone call? A meeting? How you do it is less important than what you say and that you act.

Betsy remembers:

Some friendships are just too deep and too important to let go. Vickie and I have a bond that goes back more than 35 years to my early years of marriage and motherhood. Probably because our bond is so intense—and probably because we are both outspoken and opinionated—we often have disagreements. One, however, arose over a misunderstanding, and the rift lasted for several painful years. One day, a mutual friend called to tell me that Vickie's father had died, and I wrote her a heartfelt note of sympathy. That broke the ice; she responded warmly and we met and re-established our friendship. Now, whenever we have an argument (which, I blush to say, still happens with some frequency), we both make a commitment to talk it out, however painful, and thrash out our differences. We've said on many occasions that our friendship has been through so much and has weathered so many real and imaginary storms that it should last forever! Regardless, we both have come to value our friendship on so many levels (spiritual as well as social, familial, and professional). Repeatedly, we both take risks to repair the friendship after each breach, and repeatedly our risk is rewarded with an even deeper friendship.

Be willing to take the first huge step for girlfriends who matter. Be willing to move forward without recrimination and without constant reference to the incidents of the past. Assume that you both learned something and that if you are willing to make an effort and she is willing to accept it, you have firm ground for your friendship to grow.

Embedded in the concept of risking a friendship is the myth that by being a friend you make yourself vulnerable and jeopardize your security. How wrong that is. The only myth here is that anything is secure. Nothing is given to us to keep. So, if you take a risk and accept a girlfriend into your life, you may open the door for something positive and rewarding. Will the relationship last a lifetime? No one knows. What you can be sure of though is that you are giving yourself a chance to enrich your life.

Judy recalls:

I think back to one time when the estrangement had gone on for several years. There were numerous misunderstandings, slights and old jealousies. The relationship was gradually moving towards an irrevocable place. Each holiday that passed and each birthday missed pushed it farther down the road. It took an act of courage to write to this person and to ask for understanding and forgiveness. This woman was and continues to be important to me so I knew that I would do whatever was necessary to make our friendship vital again. It took months. Letters exchanged. Then the tentative phone call and finally a meeting with tears and words of appreciation on both sides. I used to go to bed at night alternating between sadness and anger about what had happened between us. What I feel now is relief and peace and I am happy to have her back in my life.

Avoid codependency

You enter into a girlfriendship with courage when you know that you can survive without this girlfriendship if that becomes necessary to your own well-being. It is this kind of thinking that allows you to make your best decisions. To draw an analogy to the business world makes the point. We have known for a long time that one advantage some women have in the workplace is independence. No one talks about it, but if a woman is working because she wants to rather than because she has to, she may make different decisions than if she has to keep her job. In girlfriendship and in the workplace, knowing you always have the option to say goodbye means, we think, that everyone behaves better.

Women with a history of making and having trustworthy girlfriends find that when they are in crisis, girlfriends sustain them. At a time when, emotionally, you don't have the energy to create new girlfriendships, your network of girlfriends is there. The history provides a grounding and, in a sense, a girlfriend bank to draw upon in times of need. A young woman explained that her own mother was grieving as she watched her grandmother die. A lifetime with few girlfriends left the woman alone and at a time when she needed

44

support, none was there. Now she is learning, slowly, painfully, how to find a girlfriend—and she finally understands that human connectedness is at the heart of who we are.

Seek and offer support

For Judy, the lesson that some women can stand with you and some cannot came with divorce. For others, the lesson comes through illness, accidents, or problems with children. For this discussion, the inciting cause is less important than the realization. It is essential—vital—to know that the disappointment must not keep you from forming friendships again. Maybe next time you will make better choices or maybe your expectations for friendship will change—you just keep trying. You will not be able to support everyone in your life who turns to you in need, and you cannot expect everyone else to stop in their tracks to help you. Protect yourself by having many sympathetic friends and by creating a reserve of reliable friends that you can draw upon and aid in hard times. The girlfriend who will help you through your next crisis may not even be known to you now. The willingness to reach out begins in girlhood and it continues for a lifetime.

Taking risks fosters growth

Judy remembers:

I was married to a difficult person—demanding, demeaning, verbally abusive. In those days, we didn't talk often about domestic violence. Rather we said that someone had a bad temper or was hard to get along with or drank too much. It wasn't until years later and through a program that I was working on with the YWCA, that I was able to give my situation a name and to accept that I had been verbally abused. Fortunately, as the abuse

45

escalated, my ego strengthened so that before it was too late, I was able to protect my children and myself by telling my husband to leave. It was probably the hardest thing I have ever had to do. But a woman helped me in a most unusual way. Brash, opinionated, sarcastic, funny, Monica was known to me from school programs and neighborhood gatherings. I thought of her as a social acquaintance. Yet, one evening we attended the same party; I was dressed in a beautiful gown with my social mask intact, anxious because I knew my husband could be humiliating in social situations.

I was standing beside the dance floor stoically watching as he insulted a woman friend of mine, causing her to cry. I knew it would be useless to intervene. Monica quietly came to my side and said in a soft voice, "You must be made of steel." I was stunned because she understood what was going on, because she was willing to acknowledge what she was seeing, because she reached out to me when I was incapable of reaching out to anyone. She helped me through my divorce and we remained good and close friends until she died 20 years ago.

What is most important about the Monica story is that she saw that I needed help and was courageous enough to help me. Did she take a risk? Without question. Her risks ranged from my husband diverting his viciousness to her to me denying the truth and accusing her of interfering. She saw someone in trouble and she acted. Those six words from her were the foundation for what became one of the best friendships of my life.

Just know that sometimes you have to take a chance for joy, knowing that you can withstand the crests and troughs without getting seasick. Taking a risk gives you an opportunity to grow. Some of our interviewees told us that experiencing pain in one girlfriendship allowed them to appreciate the pleasure in another. The strength to take risks then, comes not from keeping strong feelings away but from knowing that you can live with them. In a good girlfriendship, you and your friend hold and nurture one another's feelings. That is what friendship means.

We hope you find the risks inherent in friendship are outweighed by the rewards to be had in an intimate, nourishing relationship that is a real girlfriendship—one that reveals to you your true and best self. May you always be willing to risk for girlfriendship and may you be well rewarded!

Ideas to think about

- To have great friendships you must be willing to explore your most vulnerable side.
- Your girlfriendships can teach you to handle failure.
- The strength to take risks comes not from keeping strong feelings away, but from knowing that you can live with heightened emotion.
- Be brave enough to find and cherish girlfriends and weave them into your life.

My thoughts

-
-
-

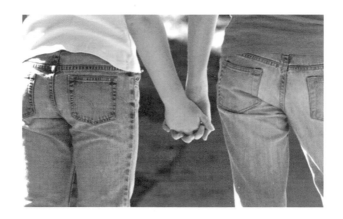

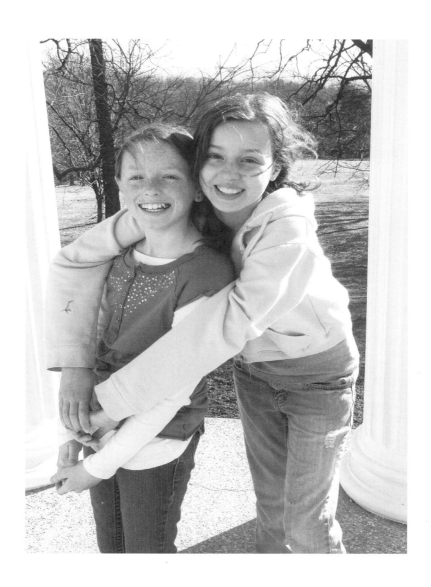

We have always loved the anonymous saying "A friend is someone who knows the song in your heart and can sing it back to you when you have forgotten the words."

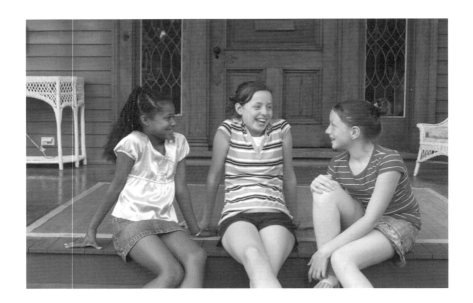

CHAPTER 4

Best Friends Forever

Now to the juicy topic of best friends—whether you have them, what they mean to you, and how necessary they are. Defining best friend is difficult because there is not one single, all encompassing description. Typically, women use words like loyal, trustworthy, helpful, dependable, kind, and caring—traits we may well expect in *all* our friends. We understand the thinking. However, what is not clear is what sets one friendship apart from others and makes it special and "best"—length of friendship? time spent together? shared interests? common problems?

Sometimes the best friend relationship seems to be forged through crises. Other women and girls like to say that they have a best friend because it announces to the world that they are lovable and someone likes them. It creates a cord of security. To our younger readers, we suggest that you be aware that you may or may not have one or more best friends in your lifetime, but the number is

51

inconsequential. The truth is that you can live happily and fully with one friend or a constellation of friends. You just need to understand yourself and what you are willing to give to a friendship and what you want in return.

When is a friend a best friend?

We use the word friend loosely to identify someone we have a relationship with—casual or expedient or devoted. Some people describe many people as friends with little attention to the differences between acquaintance and friend, friendly and friend.

Judy recounts that the distinction was made clear to her one day when she was talking with a well-known woman—a once-successful business owner, power broker, philanthropist, and hostess—who had gotten into serious trouble and later went to prison. At one point (and in tears) she asked what happened to her friends—the people who accepted her money, her party invitations, and vied to spend time with her and have their pictures taken. She had been deluded, as many of us are, thinking that these people were her friends. Rather, they were using her and as soon as she could no longer do things for them, they were gone. Her situation was dramatic, played out publicly in the media, but the message for you is this: Analyze carefully why you are friends with someone and she with you. The world is full of sycophants who might sound and look like friends, but in the last scene they are off to the next party. It is easy to be friends with someone when days are sunny, it is when trouble comes that you test your mettle and that of your friends.

Sometimes this "best" friend is one fabulous person, or in the drama of our lives, the role of best friend may be played by a changing cast of characters. There is an old saying that "Some friends are for a season, some for a reason, and some for a lifetime." A friend comes into our lives at a certain time for a certain reason, and then moves out of our lives or at least into the background. Don't begrudge or regret those "seasonal" friends. They are with us, and then they—*or we*—move on. Still, they enrich us immeasurably, since we are the sum total of all our relationships.

A group of best friends

Not all of you—or indeed all of us—can say that we have one best girlfriend. Actually, we doubt that many women do. More common and probably more possible, is the concept of a group of good friends meeting situational, emotional, and spiritual needs. Sharing time and space and then as life swirls on, moving together and apart. Think back to the inseparable girl friendships of your teenage years, your friends from summer camp, your friends from college. We believed, and imagine that you did too, that these girlfriendships were inviolate. We sang songs about eternal devotion. We talked until late in the night, we lived together and we shared each other's lives.

But as fast as we moved together, we moved apart with lingering memories, laughter and tears, and fear of loneliness.

Judy remembers:

One of my best girlfriendship experiences happened during my sophomore year at the University of Colorado. I was randomly assigned to a bedroom suite at the sorority house with four suitemates—one girl I knew from my freshman year and three other girls who had just transferred to Boulder. Our names drew us together initially—three Judys, a Julia and a Jeannie. All but one of us was from the south and all but one of us had a southern accent. Later, friends told us that no one understood a word we said for six months. A suite sounds grand but actually it was in the basement and had two bedrooms with a common bathroom and a little sitting area where our telephone was located (no cell phones then). These girls were hilarious and we laughed our way through an entire year. We shared clothes, stories, and homework. We had our own posse and if anyone had asked me then, I would have said that these four girls were my best friends. We stayed in touch for several years but gradually our lives diverged. I know where two of the girls are now and when I consider all of the people that I met in college, these four are the ones I would like to see most of all. It was the humor, I think, that made it memorable. We didn't face life-altering problems, we were not asked to make life choices. We did learn how to be together and to create girlfriendship bonds that warm me to this day.

Reviving old friendships

For each of you there are probably one, two, or three people you still connect with, years after what brought you together is over. You can pick up immediately where your conversation ended. You can still understand the shorthand that you wrote together with hours of intimacies exchanged and experiences shared. But we would argue that the continuation of the friendship rarely happens unless you can occasionally be together in person. Not just instant messages and phone conversations.

We heard from a number of women, mainly in their 50s and 60s, who have gone back and resurrected girlfriendships from the past. They have found ways to be together on a regular basis and they have enjoyed the serenity of being with people with whom they share memories and loyalty forged over many years. Someone who knew them at summer camp when a shower was only a weekly occurrence and they didn't wash their hair all summer, who visited with their parents and met their high school boyfriend, who made them laugh when divorce was coloring their world in gray and black.

We each remember times in our lives when a friendship emerged, bloomed and blossomed with a sudden intensity, and then—seemingly just as swiftly, faded. Even though they wither and die, you don't stop enjoying flowers—friends are the same!

Betsy remembers*:*

My college best friend and I enjoyed an easy sharing of our deepest plans and dreams about life. We were so close, we knew each other's very thoughts—and even after graduation we remained close. Then she married and happily immersed herself in family life, while I remained single and career-oriented for a few more years. Our friendship continued—as it does to this day—but not with the same "best friend" intensity. She and I nurture a firm bond that reaches back to that first scary day of college orientation when two shy freshmen (brought together by the Freshman Dean as "opposite types") met and began a lifelong process of mutual support.

I remember how she unwittingly cheered homesick me – as I listened at night to her sniffles (caused, I later discovered, only by allergies, not grief), I figured she was even more bereft than I felt, and was summarily and strangely comforted. She remains a steady and cheerful beacon in my life and I cherish her and our friendship.

I treasure the "best friend" of my single working years; the Mary Tyler Moore to my Rhoda. We laughed and cried our way through the singles world in San Francisco. We remember several disastrous blind dates and one hilarious Thanksgiving dinner when the turkey failed to roast on time and twenty hungry singles waited. Ours was a life-defining friendship and it too endures today, though in a less vibrant form. And let's not forget the best friends of the early marriage and child rearing years—my best friend of those years and I shared an in-the-trenches camaraderie and loyalty that rivals those war-buddy stories that emerge from every boot camp. We shared play dates and anxious waits by a child's sickbed. In each case, a best friend emerged from a life situation to support, define, and teach me, and provide for me a priceless gift, even after the relationship that created the gift had ended.

Best friends are nice but not necessary

In fact, the concept of our need for a best friend may be based on a different, less complicated society when there were fewer girlfriendship options. Women's lives in earlier times were more proscribed; they lived in the same place with the same people; fewer worked and there were fewer options for outside relationships.

Some fortunate women have been able to sustain girlfriendships over many years—with a sister or a cousin or a niece, or one in a sequence of strong and firm girlfriendships.

What these women tell us is that when they are with their girlfriend, it's as if they have never been apart. If these kinds of girlfriendships are part of your life, you can pick up right where you left off—even if it's years later.

These girlfriends share your values and ideals. They will be honest with you. They help you through rough times with your families, your work, and your lives—and they inspire you with their own great qualities. Your best friends help you to be better, stronger people than you would be otherwise.

For women, girlfriends provide support through all phases of the life cycle, raising families together and supporting each other through the traumas and triumphs of life, regardless of geographical distance. As one woman declared:

"She [my best friend] and I enjoy each other's company and strengths. We rely on those strengths to fill in where we may be weak. We share our lives; love each other's husband and children. I know she would be there for me and do anything for me as I would for her, no questions asked. We have shared the births of our children, family illnesses, deaths, moves, diets, and homes."

So what if you don't have, haven't had, might not ever have a best girlfriend? Is there something wrong with you? Of course not! You may have good girlfriends, but you may decide that you do not need or want to make one girlfriend first among equals. The decision always comes back to you and how you choose to relate to people. We believe that current lifestyles work against having one best girlfriend because life today is lived in a more fluid way. Consider that the model of the almost nomadic family is more common now than ever before. It used to be that military families were the ones that moved frequently, now it is the way of life for many of us. People change jobs every seven years and often the changes result in uprooting the family, changing schools, moving to a new neighborhood, forming new friendships. We may become wary of forming close girlfriendships because we don't want to experience the sadness that comes when the girlfriendship ends. Further, being a best friend requires time, commitment, and energy. When we are forced to leave old girlfriends behind and once again make new friendships, we become tired and stop trying so hard.

The other side of long-distance girlfriendship is that sometimes it is easier to maintain a friendship with someone who lives away because you can feel as if you have a best friend but you have more control over the time and energy that you devote to the friendship. Judy reflects about one woman she sees for four to six weeks each year. During that time, they have adventures in the most exotic places and talk about everything—probably even issues that would not be discussed with someone she sees regularly at a party on Saturday night. Yet, when it is time to go home, these two women go back to their own lives, sharing email and phone calls, but with no expectation that they are going to have holiday dinners together or lunch every Saturday. Judy thinks of this woman as one of her best friends and knows she could call her if she needed help because they care about each other. In today's mobile world, it may be that relationships with girlfriends—best friends or not—will be more similar to this.

Draw on your girlfriend bank

Do not assume that by forming a best girlfriendship, your girlfriend will be there when you need her. Much of life you will experience by yourself. But you can create what we call a girlfriend bank. And, what you ask is that? Well, in our lexicon it means that over your lifetime you have been a good friend to a few or many women and that through these relationships you have learned how to hold the feelings of another, to be kind and to be giving and honest. Not all of these women will be there when you need to draw upon your "reserve bank," but some will. And they are evidence that you know how to find and keep a friend. Using the metaphor of the circle, you will help or be helped by someone else.

Ironically, at the very times when you might need the continuity and security of best girlfriends the most—when extended family isn't there, old girlfriends may not be available. That's when the "guardian angels" step in—the phrase one midlife woman used to describe the emergency "new" best girlfriends that often show up just when needed, and when family and "real" best friends aren't available.

Betsy recalls:

I still remember with awe and gratitude the time when I was going through a very dark period, a time of a seemingly undiagnosable illness in a family member. One caring friend, whom I wouldn't have characterized as a "best" girlfriend, heard the panic and fear in my voice, came over immediately and took charge of the situation. She calmly but firmly told me what I needed to do, and even set up an appointment with her own doctor. She literally and figuratively carried me through a difficult time, and I remember her with loving gratitude today. For me, she defines what girlfriend means whether we call it "best" or not.

Avoid hurtful relationships

Know that even with good girlfriendships, the path is not always smooth. Sometimes one of you will disappoint the other; but a good girlfriendship is one where you both are willing to accept both sadness and joy and go forward. But the girlfriendship based upon competition and envy is, as one woman told us, toxic. Another woman explained that for many years she actually had betrayal dreams—nightmares with knives and backstabbing women.

One woman, call her Linda, told us about a situation that happened to her. She moved to a large city to be with the man she was planning to marry. A woman in the man's circle of friends befriended her. Asked her to dinner. Made theatre plans. Acted like a caring and thoughtful girlfriend. It took a few months for Linda to find out that the friendship was a ruse and that each time the two women were together, a third woman had a date with the fiancé. Bad behavior all around. Hurtful. Duplicitous. Dishonest. Truly toxic.

You can learn about a girlfriend by watching how she treats others. Don't be fooled thinking that there is something special about you and that you won't be treated that way—you will. If you don't like who you are when you with this person, stay away. You don't change people. Either you interact with them in a healthy, loving, mutually beneficial way or you accept that this person is not your girlfriend. A twelve year old put it best:

"If you tell a secret to one of your BFF's (best friends forever) and they tell it to everybody without your permission, then that is not your BFF."

Become your own best girlfriend

Sometimes, you become your own best girlfriend. That's right; remember what you already know deep down about yourself: that you are a valuable, unique person who deserves the best that life has to offer. You are an amazing and beautiful woman with so much to give back to the world. You have to remind yourself of your good qualities and cheer yourself up even if you think that you have failed. In short, you have to provide yourself with the nurture and support of a best girlfriend—and your very ability to do that for yourself is your strength, and a proof of your growing independence. In fact, your ability to survive and thrive without a traditional "best friend" may even be your own best qualification for friendship! (Ironic isn't it?) To be strong and centered enough to live without a best girlfriend makes you more apt to have one!

In fact, the whole notion of having a "best" friend may reflect an insecurity on our part. Think back to elementary school and junior high school; wasn't the eagerness to "have" a "best friend forever" a reflection of your need to belong, to have a secure emotional place in the confusion of adolescence? In the end, what really matters is your own sense of the "rightness" of where you search for and find emotional support.

Remember that, although we all like to say that we have a best girlfriend, it's the *friend* part that matters not the *best* part. Having good girlfriends is important; having best girlfriends is not always possible, but remember what Toni Morrison said best, "the loneliest woman in the world is the woman without a close woman friend."

Ideas to think about

- A girlfriend bank will sustain you over a lifetime.
- First, you have to be your own best girlfriend.
- It's the *friend* part that matters, not the *best*.

My thoughts

-
-
-

61

Girlfriends do not substitute for family, rather— chosen carefully and tended lovingly—girlfriends can create a new extended family.

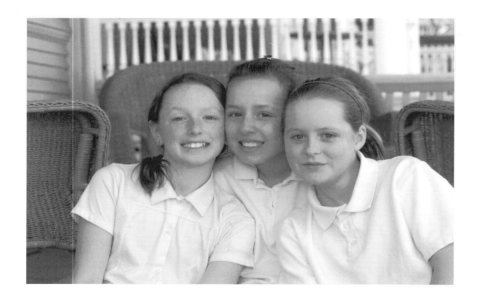

Chapter 5

Friends as Family

Well, here it is—the question that causes endless hours of angst and generates enough guilt for Woody Allen. Basically, you ask yourself—as we have before you—do I have to choose between my girlfriends and my family?

How you answer this question for yourself provides guidance for everything that you do. We believe, and hope that you agree, that both girlfriends and family are important and that one does not substitute for another. Rather, it is possible to achieve a balance so that your life is enriched by both girlfriends and family. In a perfect world, girlfriends can become like family and your mothers, your sisters, your aunts can be girlfriends.

The point is to have great people in your life whether they are part of your family or not. The choice should not be made based on biology, but rather common interests, caring, kindness, and integrity.

Judy Remembers:

I have often thought that summer camp is a place where the role of family and friend intersect in an important way.

My own experience is an example. Each summer for many years I went away to a small summer camp in North Carolina. Each year my parents would drive my sisters and me to camp and each year I would dread the day we were going. I stopped sleeping. I was frightened. I didn't want to go. But, staying home was not an option.

So, we packed up and off we went. My sisters loved camp and to this day, one of them sees it as the best experience of her life. I, on the other hand, cried when my parents left and felt desolate for days after. Sundays were the worst. But slowly, I began to make friends or found friends from years past. I discovered things to enjoy—the horseback riding, the crafts shop, activities after dinner. (I never liked swimming at 7:30 a.m. in the cold pool fed by mountain streams and I never liked hiking up and down the hills to get there).

But I adjusted and by the time the six weeks had ended and my parents were back to pick us up, I cried again. Why? Because I had to leave camp and my friends and the horses and the homemade biscuits. What else? The independence and the joy in feeling that I was able to live outside of my safe and secure family group. In a sense, over that time period, the girlfriends and the counselors became my family. The transition was always painful, but I learned that I could move from my family to a larger world and I learned how to interact with people to make that a good experience.

How does this relate to forming girlfriendships? Well, summer camp showed me that on my own and without my family, I could not just survive but actually enjoy relationships with other people. It showed me that I didn't have to choose one or the other, but could move within both worlds. It provided a relatively safe environment for me to test what I was learning at home and to try to choose those girls who would be good and trusted friends.

What we want to know

Let us think about how girlfriends and family fit together in your life, what your girlfriends bring to your life that your family doesn't—or can't—and how relationships between you and your family are different than those between you and your girlfriends.

What women told us

We posed these questions to many women of varying ages. From many we heard that girlfriends bring a less judgmental point of view than family. Their girlfriendships were often based on mutual interest and need.

You may find this to be true. You often have more flexibility in a girlfriendship than with family members because with girlfriends you always have the option to say goodbye in a way that is far different from ending a relationship with your mother or your sister.

Girlfriends bring a different perspective to our lives. They come without your personal family baggage and they fill in where family cannot. For instance, in some families, feelings are discussed and are part of the family fabric. In others, that is not true. You will find yourself consciously and unconsciously searching for what is missing in your life. It can be something as simple as finding someone who likes to go to basketball games or shop for handbags. Or it can be at a different level when you want to find someone who will be honest about how you are handling a family problem or the breakup with a boyfriend.

One young woman told us: "My girlfriends are concerned about me like my family, but are more likely to point out how I could have done better in assessing or handling a situation."

Inspired by a memory, Betsy wrote this note to her daughter Bess: *As my mother—your wise grandmother—used to say (long before I understood the truth in what she said): "You can pick your friends, but you inherit your family."*

Balancing girlfriends and family

Girlfriends can allow you to see different aspects of yourself that your family may not appreciate or see. They can bring objectivity and a degree of separation that is impossible with family. Girlfriends can help you make sense of family dynamics. And, girlfriendships have another more subtle role in your life—they can help you understand that you can survive failure. A strange statement? Think about it carefully.

Not all of your girlfriendships are going to lead to lifelong relationships. You may be disappointed by a girlfriend or she by you. Betrayal? Dishonesty? Disregard for feelings? You might be hurt but, you will learn—if you haven't already—that you can gather yourself together and go on. It is important to have that resource within yourself for the difficult times ahead.

When balancing girlfriends and family, the element of choice is primary, but close behind is history and common experiences. Your relationships with your family are bound with ties that can allow you to feel secure and valued, but also constricted. You have the natural connections that allow relationships to continue. But still you will find that there are times when what you need is your dearest girlfriend even if you adore your family. You build a family structure apart from that which you knew as a child.

One of Judy's granddaughters put it best when she was five years old and Judy told her that she had loved her from the moment she was born. The child replied, "Well then, who loved me before I was born?"

We do not believe that girlfriends substitute for family, rather, chosen carefully and tended lovingly, girlfriends can be an extended family. You may find girlfriends whom you like better than some members of your family, but that doesn't mean that you discard either one.

One woman, describing how someone had helped her explained: "It was my sister, which is not the same thing as a friend."

What could and should happen is that the relationships complement one another. Families do not have to be friends, likewise girlfriends do not have to be family. The choices are yours.

Sometimes in practical ways, girlfriends are family. You and your family live far from one another. You talk on the phone and send messages and visit now and then, but for most of the days of the year, your family is not there. What this means is that you begin to fill the void. Where do you have Thanksgiving dinner? Who is going to be invited to your daughter's birthday party? Who can pick you up at the doctor's office when you can't drive yourself home? You turn to girlfriends and over time, they begin to function as a surrogate family for you and you for them.

Judy's example for her daughters:

I remember how you experienced friends becoming temporary family. When you were children, we lived on a small street with two other families, a total of nine children. None of us had extended family living in the same city. As you girls grew up, you became close to the other two families. You spent the night together, you ate together, you celebrated big events together, you had street carnivals to raise money for the cancer fund—you even had arguments as sisters do.

In many ways, your friends became your family. We were family for each other. None of us abandoned our real families; indeed, the familial ties were as strong as ever. But we were there when the real family couldn't be.

But here is where the difference between family and friends is most apparent. More than 20 years has passed since the last of the nine children graduated from high school. One family moved. Contact is limited. Memories are left. Several years ago, one of their daughters returned to Cincinnati for a class reunion. We had lunch.

This girl ate with us, slept with us, spent many days and weeks at our house. Yet, here we were sitting in a restaurant making small talk and having lunch looking at pictures of her children. We had tears in our eyes because we understood that what was gone couldn't be recovered. But, we agreed, we wouldn't have missed the friendship experience just because it would end. We learned. We grew. We had fun and our memories will last until we die.

With your real family, communication and contact most often continue even when circumstances change. With girlfriends that is not always true.

Lifelong or ephemeral relationships

You could draw a conclusion that girlfriends come to be surrogate families to meet mutual needs while real families are together because they are, simply put, family. With real family come responsibilities, obligations, and expectation of lifelong relationships.

It is in this context that your girlfriendships live and where the tension between girlfriendships and family relationships is strong.

We yearn for history

As we grow older and our world begins to shrink, we find that we begin to think of our girlfriends in a new and important way. As women age, most of us yearn for history, for connections with people we knew when we were young, who knew some of the same people that we remember fondly.

Many older women confirmed for us that it is easy to be dismissive of family and girlfriends when you are 35 and your horizons stretch forever. But when you are 60, the world looks different. This message was not surprising but was compelling in its consistency:

- Value your girlfriendships and your families.
- Honor and relive your history.
- Remember that girlfriends can help stave off the specter of aloneness.

Our daughters and young readers may not understand these words now, but at a juncture—different for everyone—family and girlfriends begin to blend. The family ties create a natural connection, but as you age, you will search for people who understand you, who can hold your feelings whether they are part of your real family or not.

Family connections

None of this precludes, of course, close relationships between family members. Many of you may find that your sister is your best friend. At a minimum, you share the family secrets. But your family connection is not inviolate. You have choices about how to be connected later in life. Fortunate are those who can truthfully say, "My daughter says that I am her best friend and I feel the same about her."

Sometimes we think that relationships with our family are less risky than those with someone unrelated to us. That is not always true. Families can make demands that friends never would. And, in fairness, we can be the one making the demands rather than receiving them.

We believe that the historical function of the family changes as young adults move away and establish lives somewhere else. In the past, families were present physically. More time was spent during the day nurturing family relationships. If one person in your family couldn't help you, another one could. The extended family that had known you since birth served as aunts, surrogate mothers, and girlfriends. For many of us, that world is gone and we look for other connections to provide joy and understanding and, when necessary, to relieve the pain of isolation and loneliness.

As mothers, we admit to seeing the relationships between mothers and daughters as emblematic of family and we believe that for each of you, your relationship with your mother encapsulates your family experiences in the most intense way. In the best of worlds, your mothers—indeed all mothers—teach daughters how to be girlfriends and demonstrate why human connection is important. Mothers can give their daughters confidence to venture forth and to take risks. With them, one learns the meaning of trust.

Sometimes we need buffers *from* our mothers and other family members. Too often the roles we had as children persist into adulthood. As children, those with siblings vied for parental attention and developed behavior patterns that became the foundation of their personalities. Does this dynamic work for or against the evolution of a sisterhood into a girlfriendship? The question has not been answered. Girlfriends can help to provide distance from your family when you need it. Girlfriends can be confidants, sounding boards, and playmates.

What women told us

We considered the responses of our group of women and attempted to discern common threads; we found several. First, and this comes as no surprise, there is not unanimity about the role of the family versus the role of the girlfriend. Obviously, family constellations differ. However, what we did find is greater agreement about the role of the family relative to the age of the women.

- For the youngest girls, family was seen as central to their world because they are dependent upon their family and often the best relationships up to that point in their lives have been with family members.
- Older women spoke of the reality of both family and girlfriends disappearing one by one, their circle growing smaller. Until, at the end of life, often only girlfriends are left. They may be girlfriends from childhood or girlfriendships newly made. One woman succinctly told us: "My girlfriends have become my family."

Friends are a tonic

A recent article in a British medical journal (J Epideiol, *Community Health* 2005; 59: 538-9) reported that a network of good friends, rather than close family ties, helps you live longer in older age because friends may influence health behaviors, such as smoking and drinking, or seeking medical help for troubling symptoms. Friends may also have important effects on mood, self-esteem, and coping mechanisms in times of difficulty.

As we heard from almost 100 women and girls, we became convinced that the relationships among girlfriends and family was not and did not need to be either/or. Relationships could, and perhaps should, be *and*. We agree with the woman who accurately told us that girlfriends do not substitute for family, they complement each other.

Our message to our daughters and readers:

Be willing to accept girlfriends as your family when the need or the opportunity presents itself. Look for the sister you never had, the mother who has died or lives far away. You can have both in your life—girlfriends and family—they are not mutually exclusive. Just know that even though you may be asked to choose one over the other because of conflicting needs or demands, compromise and resolution are possible—and welcome.

Be brave enough to find and cherish girlfriends and weave them into your life. Our families and our friend-families—large and small, nuclear and extended—nourish us. It is not an accident that girlfriends are often called "sisters" without the existence of a familial relationship.

Cincinnati poet Annie Ruth put it best. "Sisterhood is essential for the soul. I was taught to be a sister and being a sister draws sisters to me. To truly embrace sisterhood in its fullness, we must first become the sisters that we yearn to have in our lives. . . "

Sister

The magnitude of her strength
Is not determined by age, relation, or gene.
She supersedes womb or seed.
Mentor, friend, and confidant.
She is endurance, fortitude, and strength.

Annie Ruth

Ideas to think about

- Girlfriends can support, define, and encourage you in ways that your family cannot.
- Girlfriends do not substitute for family, rather, chosen carefully and tended lovingly, girlfriends can create a new extended family.
- The point is to have great people in your life whether they are part of your family or not.
- You have more flexibility in a girlfriendship because with girlfriends you have the option to say goodbye in a way far different from ending a relationship with your mother or your sister.

My thoughts

-
-
-

As we realize that we are near the start of the end of our lives, we search for those who knew us, who understood us, who validate that our life has had meaning.

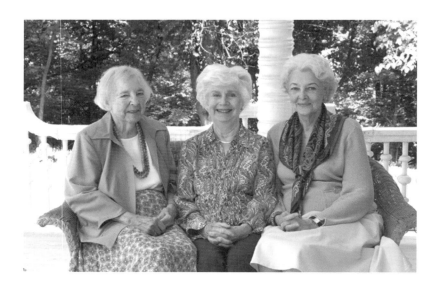

CHAPTER 6

Only the History

As we move through the passages of our lives, our relationships change. That is not a revolutionary statement but it is important to remember especially when you are considering your girlfriendships and what they have meant to you.

A girlfriendship that seemed inviolate and forever when you were in college, may feel like an empty exercise now. The same woman you couldn't wait to talk to is one with whom you now have trouble making conversation. You stretch for the past and for common interest and find it without life and color. You fear that she feels the same way and you worry about your ability to sustain girlfriendships, to be a good and loyal girlfriend, to neither use nor feel used.

In fact, if you are like us, you blame yourself for your inability to sustain a friendship. We want to assure you that the emotion you feel around this girlfriendship is not only common but the norm. You will meet few people with whom you can maintain a girlfriendship over extended years and through many life changes. Most of your girlfriendships will be ones that are intense and focused on the situation you both find yourselves in—the college dormitory, the preschool class, and the dinner club. But then you graduate from college, your children grow up, your dinner club disbands, your interests change, and you move on. Others, those that are more profound, are based on a feeling of affinity, which may spring from a long history or a single meeting.

Judy recalls:

Probably the person who best captures for me the essence of short but intense and important friendships is a tall, creative woman whose life work is creating beautiful clothing and imparting serenity. When you are in her presence or in her clothes you feel comforted, warm, and beautiful. Lovely soft fabrics that float, small details like little crystals and beads (sewn inside a cuff or under a collar) that only you can see, unusual ways of wrapping and folding that turn a scarf into a jacket and a dress into a cocoon. All reflective of her interest in you as a person. I met this woman about ten years ago and although we have never lived in the same city and I have only seen her in person once, I still think of her as friend. We send cards and letters. Sometimes we talk by phone, but every time I open my closet and select something that she designed for me, I know she is close. I could call her if I was in trouble and she would come. I could tell her that I was depressed and her soothing words would lift my spirits. I can tell her the truth and not feel judged. Friendship? I think so.

Celebrate the temporary

What we want to emphasize is this: girlfriendships have value for you and for your girlfriends even when they are limited in time and space. We call it celebrating the temporary and at its essence, it means that it is important to value what you have now, to take the risks that girlfriendship involves and to be grateful for today because tomorrow may be different. We can assure you that tomorrow *will* be different, but what you shared becomes a part your soul and your personality.

During your lifetime you will continue to develop new girlfriendships. Be open to them. And recognize that over the years, you may choose—or your girlfriend may choose—to come back and to work to rebuild a girlfriendship that seemed lost. The history allows girlfriendship to reopen but the future will be based on what you have in common. It is worthwhile to make the effort to keep your girlfriendships alive.

The shared history

You understand the feelings. You go to a party or a reunion or you accidentally encounter a girlfriend from your past—within a few minutes the time has been erased and you are talking and laughing and reminiscing about what happened months or years before. This is the girlfriend who remembers that your mother told her mother that high school senior girls were rendered so obnoxious, that when they left for college, it was less painful, who knew that your incredibly blonde college roommate had to paint on her face every day, who was there when your mother found out that one of your friends had climbed into the clothes dryer and broken it.

The question for you is this: does the initial excitement lead either one of you to seek further contact or does the frisson die down and you part with a limp goodbye and a promise to call sometime to schedule lunch? Obviously, there is not one answer. Just know that as you grow older, the early contacts and the history become valuable to you in a way you probably cannot understand while in your 20s. Women in their 50s and 60s told us that forming new girlfriendships takes energy: they grow tired of explaining who they are—like social job interviews. Rather, they luxuriated in the comfort and warmth of the familiar and the bonds of trust forged long before.

Betsy remembers:

I had the happiest of friendship experiences three years ago. Attending a nephew's wedding, I encountered the woman who had been my very best friend from the first through the fifth grade (a time when best friends seem crucial to life) when she abruptly left our school for another and effectively vanished from my small young orbit. I had been devastated at the time, and had (subconsciously) mourned her loss all these years. What a thrill to encounter her again! Did she remember me? Did she feel the same way? Had she wondered about me all these years? Half apprehensively, like girls simultaneously dreading and longing for a blind date, we scheduled a luncheon get together. And what a revelation it was!

Words poured out of both of us as we tried to fill all the gaps of those lost years. We had so much to catch up on and, although our lives had taken different paths (she had married and had children earlier than I did and had lived in Europe with her family). We found much in common. She was still the same—loyal and dear and sympathetic, but wise and sharp and funny as well. Joyfully, we reconnected and vowed to keep in touch. And so we have, meeting frequently for lunches or visits, talking often on the phone. And each time we come together, we are grateful, remembering what a gift it is to rediscover a lost childhood friendship in adulthood and recognize the girls we were in the women we have become.

Childhood friends know who we were

From many older women we heard a frequent refrain. As they have aged, these women have begun to feel a longing to talk with people who knew them when they were younger. They seek out their old girlfriends to determine whether there is a path to close girlfriendship again. They build on what existed before. It may be that as we realize that we are near the start of the end of our lives, we search for those who knew us, who understood us, who validate that our life has had meaning. Someone who can acknowledge not only who we are but also who we were.

Frequently we heard from women in their 60s who:

- Yearn for girlfriends who are gone either by relocation or death or a break in the relationship.
- Try to reconnect and welcome people from the past to spend time with the "me of today."
- Know that girlfriendships that last a lifetime may not be common but treasure those girlfriendships when they have them.
- Understand that someone who is a girlfriend at one time may become a girlfriend again later in life.
- Are aware that reunions like partings are not always well made.

One woman, who went to boarding school, explained that she formed a lifelong girlfriendship with her roommate: "we are close to this day and travel together. I was lonely in boarding school and she was an anchor for me in a very unfamiliar and sometimes difficult environment."

We asked ourselves, does the intensity of the original girlfriendship bond predict whether the relationship can continue through the years, regardless of time and place and circumstance?

A woman in her 50s described coming together for a funeral with girlfriends from childhood. These women who had been good friends as young girls agreed to deliberately carve out time each year to take a week-long vacation together. They live in different cities but they come together annually to celebrate what they had as young women and to forge girlfriendships anew as their lives draw to a close. Obviously, what they had experienced together was strong enough to draw them together again.

Judy remembers that the idea was brought home recently when she lunched with two women she has known for more than 40 years. (She was out doing an interview for this book when she literally ran into one of the women visiting her terminally ill mother in a nursing home.)

Judy recalls:

This woman and I had been wonderful friends at several stages of our lives—college, young adults, young mothers, and community volunteers. The connection has always been there but contact has been infrequent. We live in the same city, but we haven't seen one another more than once or twice a year for 25 years. Our interests and our commitments are different. Our lives are divergent.

We scheduled a lunch date for the two of us and another mutual friend. I happily looked forward to the meeting. I wasn't disappointed. Most sentences began with "Do you remember?" or "I remember when" or "Can you believe?" There was sincere interest on all sides about our lives, our children, our history, our girlfriendship. We left the restaurant understanding how fortunate we were to be able to reconnect before it was too late. At my age I have begun to read the obituary column every day and I always find someone I know. These women are important to me and I to them.

Our message to our daughters and our readers is, "do not wait until it is too late to talk."

Our history helps to define who we are

Sometimes former girlfriends are able to connect, but that is not always so. If you are spending time with a girlfriend you have known for years but you find yourself hesitating to make plans, creating excuses or appearing at lunch wishing you were somewhere else, you need to look clearly at whether the girlfriendship is working for you or your girlfriend. Maybe in the past you have shared experiences, but no longer and not today. The question then is what to do without feeling guilty or unkind? It has happened to us more than once and we have each chosen to react in a different way.

Judy relates:

There is a group of women I have known since the early days of marriage when we learned together about being wives and later mothers. We shared recipes and dinner parties, football weekends, and visits from parents. We had plans together on most weekends, bridge and golf games during the week. We were a group, a clique, a posse and we talked on the phone every day. This went on for years, until slowly we moved to different parts of town, our children developed new friends, our personal interests changed. One woman became a preschool teacher; another divorced and got a fulltime job; another's husband became quite ill; another's

81

husband died and she remarried—common occurrences all. I went back to graduate school and later divorced. I began to develop my career and between work and the children, little time was left for the lunches, the parties, and tennis and golf games.

When I remarried and reached out again for these old friends, they weren't there. Or, put differently, they were there but not in a way that could connect with me. They were doing what we used to do and I had moved away. When my husband and I went to one of their parties, it was acutely uncomfortable because after we asked about the children and other small talk, there was nothing left to say. We began to refuse invitations and soon, they stopped coming.

So, for me, the solution was to gradually move away. There were no arguments or pronouncements, just diminished contact until there was none at all.

Recently, one of the women called me with an urgent need for an especially delicious cookie recipe. Of course, I gave it to her and we chatted for a few minutes about the old days. She told me about a mutual friend who had been recently diagnosed with cancer and about her children, now adults, coming for the holidays. She couldn't understand why I was still working and when I explained that I felt incredibly fortunate, her response was "Oh." It was nice to hear from her, but I knew as the phone call ended that we wouldn't be talking again any time soon.

Betsy reveals:

One way to end a girlfriendship is to let it die a gradual death, as in Judy's two examples. But for some people, confrontation (or as they would describe it being truthful) is a choice.

One woman, who had been a close friend of my early married years, went through an ugly, public, painful divorce, and her

82

financial circumstances changed drastically. I supported her throughout this dark period, offering a listening ear and whatever comfort I could provide. Gradually, I sensed her growing discomfort when we were together, but blindly I persisted in offering friendship, hoping we could continue as before. So I was totally unprepared one day when she bluntly told me that we could not be friends any more because I was "too demanding" of her. I was crushed and devastated, and, of course, blamed myself for the loss of the friendship. But I really didn't understand what I had done wrong. Finally, I came to realize (with the help of other good friends who were aware of the situation) that the problem lay with her—her discomfort at being around me was because I unwittingly reminded her of her previous lost life. I was a painful souvenir of something she had to move away from. It was a sad incident, and I regret it to this day. Perhaps someday we will be able to reconnect, but I doubt it.

Letting go is a part of girlfriendship

The point of these anecdotes is this: someday you will probably be either the perpetrator or the recipient of the ending of a girlfriendship. If the ending is gradual and graceful, no harm is done. If it is direct and confrontational, try not to be bitter, but to learn from it. Try to understand, not only your side (and whether you honestly wronged your friend) but hers as well. Did she need to do this for her own sake? Always there are lessons to be learned—and always the possibility of new and better girlfriendships ahead.

Not all former girlfriendships should be resurrected—nor can they be. Consider the girls you were close to in high school or college. If they appeared in your life today, would you choose them as friends? Sometimes yes. Sometimes no. But you did share something incredibly powerful and important. Anyone who has attended a class reunion understands. There is the strength of an age-old bond and common experience, but there is also the feeling of being mired in time without recognition of growth, change, and accomplishments. You don't want to go back to that, but rather, you want to be with women who can appreciate the new you with kindness and caring for what you are today and where you have been. If a girlfriend was with you in the past, that is exceptional. But, it is also possible to have outstanding girlfriendships with new girlfriends who value who you are today, without the shared history.

You will know when a girlfriendship is over or should be. And be prepared for grieving especially if it is a girlfriendship you would like to continue. If a woman has been important in your life, saying goodbye leaves a void and often an incredibly sick feeling in your stomach—a visceral, physical longing, and sadness. But letting go is as much a part of girlfriendship as forming the relationship initially. Sometimes girlfriendships just gradually end as both women drift into new patterns with new people. There seems to be almost mutual acknowledgement that the need for the girlfriendship has ended and, without bad feelings, two people separate. There may be attempts to preserve a vestige of the nostalgic bond, but frequently that bond frays and each woman goes her separate way.

Judy's example:

Let me give you an example of a personal experience that mirrors, we believe, reality for many. A long-time neighbor moved thousands of miles away. This woman had been close to me.

We walked our dogs together two miles every day. We talked on the phone often. Our children played together. We celebrated holidays together. We shared intimate thoughts and trusted one another. When she left I cried, not just that day but for days after. She told me that we would always be friends and I told her that I would always value our girlfriendship, but that once she moved the relationship would change and that we wouldn't be girlfriends in the same way again. We would both try for a while, but at some point, trying would become too hard. She didn't agree, but I knew I was right. Once the daily contact and easy sharing of thoughts were gone, so was the girlfriendship. I don't denigrate nor diminish the girlfriendship we had and I value it to this day. But we are no longer close parts of one another's lives. We have only seen each other for a few hours since she left eleven years ago; she sends Christmas letters with pictures of the children and life goes on. If we were neighbors again, we could renew our girlfriendship, but distance and lack of contact means that, for now, what we had is what there is.

Betsy writes of friendship's challenges

While speaking of lost friendships, we would be less than candid if we didn't 'fess up to the times we have failed our friends. After all, if friendship is a two-way street, sometimes the blocked traffic lies on my side of the street!

I recall with painful clarity the time that a close friend tried to confide the hurt of a broken marriage to me and I just didn't want to listen—probably because I didn't want to know the sad truth and partly because I just didn't know how to handle it. There have been other times when my pride, impatience, or just-plain-busyness prevented me from being available to my friends.

What would I do differently if I were starting over with my friends? I would be more honest (when appropriate), and more giving and forgiving—accepting my friends faults, moods, and sheer human nature while ignoring the little irritants that are part of the wonderful but challenging package of friendship.

Judy recalls not always being the good friend

It is not always easy to be a good friend, and there have been times when I failed. One example haunts me still: A woman I had known since college developed a debilitating illness and was confined to a wheelchair; she needed help. Other than scheduling a few lunch dates, I avoided her. I rationalized that I was too busy, the children needed me, and that being in the middle of a divorce myself, I simply did not have the energy to take on someone else's problems. This happened 25 years ago and I still feel embarrassed about my behavior. Being a good friend sometimes demands more than we are willing—or able—to give.

Reflect upon your memories

It is important for you to think carefully about your girlfriendships. Consider how they began, how they ended. Or, put differently, why and how have your girlfriendships disintegrated—if they have. You will answer these questions for yourself as you probe your inner thoughts to find out what attributes attracted your attention and what pathways have led to strong girlfriendships for you.

Ideas to Think About

- There are few people in a lifetime with which you can maintain a girlfriendship over many years and through many life changes.

86

- Girlfriendships have value for you and for your girlfriends even when they are limited in time and space. We call it celebrating the temporary.
- Letting go is as much a part of girlfriendship as forming the relationship initially.
- Not all former girlfriendships should be resurrected—nor can they be.

My thoughts

-

-

-

-

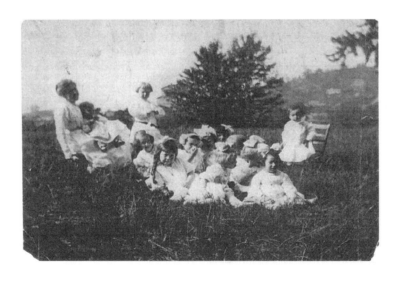

Friendships define us as women throughout our lives, but most effectively and dramatically at life's beginning and end.

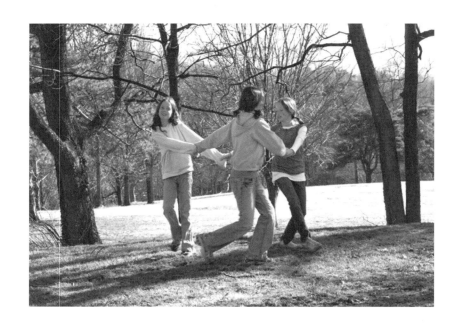

CHAPTER 7

What the Circle Teaches

As we close this book, we sense a closing of the circle. We began our study as a celebration of women's friendships and their life-enhancing qualities. We wanted to equip you—our daughters, granddaughters, and readers—with the means to deal with the joys, the risks, and the losses of friendships—and with the courage to keep trying again. In this book, we have tried to explain the ways in which friendships define us as women throughout our lives, but most effectively and dramatically at life's beginning and end.

Now we feel a need to sum up the accumulated wisdom we've derived from our interviews with the representative women who shared their thoughts on the subject of girlfriendship. As we talked with (and read the comments of) the girls and women participating in our informal survey, we were struck by the similarities of the experiences and the insights they shared.

We thought it would be instructive to share with you their unedited thoughts on the subjects we've discussed. A selection of the responses follows. Here they are—in their own voices—speaking on the girlfriendship lessons in each of our chapters.

Celebrating girlfriendships

Don't try to be someone else; just be yourself. Don't try too hard to fit in. They will like you just the way you are.
—*11 years old, private school student*

You just have to be brave and introduce yourself. If they are total snobs, they might use you for a while but if not, it is pretty easy to be friends. Don't choose friends by presence or beauty, choose by trust and personality.
—*11 years old, private school student*

Balance. Friendship is about unconditional love and mutual respect. Without the balance on both sides, there is nothing.
—*68 years old, Ph.D., widow, and professional*

You have to be yourself and if they don't like how you act, then they are not worth your time. You should not try to be someone you're not.
—*16 years old, public school student*

Girlfriends are to be selected carefully and wisely. They should energize you and not make you feel worse about yourself or your life. They can teach you how to have difficult conversations while still being able to retain a relationship. A healthy girlfriendship will enhance your relationship with your spouse because it relieves pressure from his needing to be all things for you.

—30-something, professional

I look for girlfriends who are like artists in their understanding of experience. . . and they have been guides to me in important passages in my life.

—63 years old, professional

Friendship changes over time

Sometimes it can be hard to let women into your life to be your close friends, but when you find the right ones, it's worth it. It is important to find girlfriends who have similar goals to yours even if, outwardly, they might not seem exactly the same as you.

—23 years old, single, student

Girlfriendships breathe life into your life.

—24 years old, graduate student

Cherish and protect your friendships. They should be considered one of your most valuable assets and treated as such. You can't make friends *after* you need them.

—58 years old, single, retiree

Friendship is a beautiful feeling.

—94 years old

Don't expect your friends to make up for something you are lacking. Only you can fill the voids in your life by doing something, contributing something, learning something that is meaningful to you. That said, friendships are crucial.

—63 years old, professional

Choose to live with passion

Experience the complexity of all types of friends: those who are challenging or rewarding or stimulating or boring; those who are supportive or neglectful or hurtful, those who share your beliefs or are opposed to them; those who keep confidences or those who do not; those whose glass is always half full or those whose is half empty. Embrace the risks of forming friendships. Practice, practice, practice! Grow a durable sense of humor.

—62 years old, married, scientist

Be very careful. Give yourself time before you welcome a person into your circle. Always notice how a person treats others. This will give you an idea about how they will treat you as a person.

—69 years old, volunteer

It takes a lot of work to be a good friend. If you are doing all the taking, you're not being a friend and may need to examine your motives and your relationships.

—53 years old, married, professional

I would say that strong friendships are the result of friends truly being able to be themselves, open and honest with each other, and, even if it is difficult, not letting disagreements get out of hand but rather bringing them into the open and discussing them. A good friendship is one characterized by equality—perhaps not in perfect balance on a day to day basis, but equal over the long haul. Friends help one another to grow.

—68 years old, Ph.D., widowed professional

Girlfriendships can sustain you or tear you apart. Choose carefully and wisely. Good, bad or indifferent, you will learn from your girlfriendships as you proceed along life's path.

—59 years old, married, professional

Best friends forever

It is not important how many friends you have, but the depth of the friendships matter.

—63 years old, professional

A girlfriend who is a real soul mate shares your life's joys and sorrows and this sharing deepens the reality of your own life experiences. You can learn how to "listen" to each other—that is such a gift for each person's unique personal growth.

—65 years old, volunteer

You have to be able to express yourself in full. A true friend will tell you the truth, no matter what.

—16 years old, student

It is great to have a variety of girlfriends that you relate to in different areas of your life but it is also fulfilling to have one or two friends who are there for you for the long haul and who are well matched on emotional needs and ability to provide support.

—40 years old, Ph.D.

To have a good friend, you need to learn to be a good friend. Go slowly. Shared experiences will help reveal the quality relationships that may stand the test of time.

—59 years old, married, professional

Friends and family

Girlfriends provide emotional support. And, in the end, we will be the ones left as women tend to live longer than men. At this stage, they become family.

—64 years old, married, professional, volunteer

Having girlfriends can give you an identity all your own.

—58 years old, retired, married

You discover yourself and develop perspective through friendships with women. One's friends and the honesty and strength of the friendships reveal your character.

—62 years old, married scientist

Don't act possessive; be willing to share your friendship. Girlfriends bring objectivity and a degree of separation that is impossible with family. They are essential to me to help understand and make sense out of family dynamics. And they can actually increase the amount of joy as well as bear the sorrows of family.

—65 years old, volunteer

My girlfriends are a special family.

—24 years old, graduate student

Only the history

Value friendship, value your friends. Be there for them—trying always to understand their perspective and approach to life, even if it is not always your way. Don't be afraid to disagree, but never do so by way of character assassination. If you can be a friend, you will create a web of friendships that will sustain you for your life. However, even a close friendship may not prove to be good for you at a certain point in your life, especially if it makes you feel bad about yourself. Be thoughtful, but trust your instincts.

—68 years old, Ph.D., widowed professional

If your friends are acting like they don't want to be friends anymore, don't try to change their minds. You will find new friends, don't worry.

—14 years old, student

Girlfriendships will change throughout life in both quality and quantity. Value them for what they are and don't force them into what they are not.

—31 years old, married, Ph.D.

There are times when friends disappear from your life for whatever reason. Always welcome them back when they return. And remember that listening, truly listening, to your friends are the most important thing that you can do.

—58 years old, single, retired

Friendships can change with time and may even end. But this doesn't mean that the friendship wasn't true or meaningful.

—30-something, professional

Our celebration ends and yours begins

So we end our celebration of the amazing, powerful bond of friendships, the unique sustaining thread that follows us through life. At the beginning of life our girlfriends help define us; at life's end, they are there to witness and validate our lives. Science constantly reminds us of the physical and psychic advantages provided by friends, but we don't need science to prove the obvious: we feel and act better when connected and encouraged by our friends. We wish you, our daughters, our family and readers alike, the joy and comfort of lasting friendships.

And we suggest that you, after finishing our book take time to reflect on and celebrate the current and past friendships that have nurtured you and made you whom you are today. We hope we have inspired you in at least some way to treasure, celebrate, and nurture your ever-widening circle of friends.

To you we send our love,

Betsy and Judy

P.S. The survey forms appear in the appendix, which follows. Feel free to copy them, respond to the questions, and share them with your girlfriends and family friends.

The Friendship

Extend your hand
toward me.
I would like to
offer my honest feelings
for exchange
toward your friendship.

Friendship is
a magnificent feeling—
special when you find that
gift in time.

Celebrate your life
by sharing that
treasure,
because life
begins—and ends—with
Girlfriends.

Esther Lucky
Cedar Village
April 2007

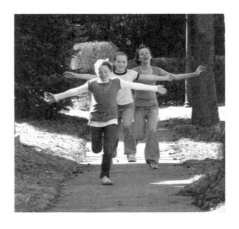

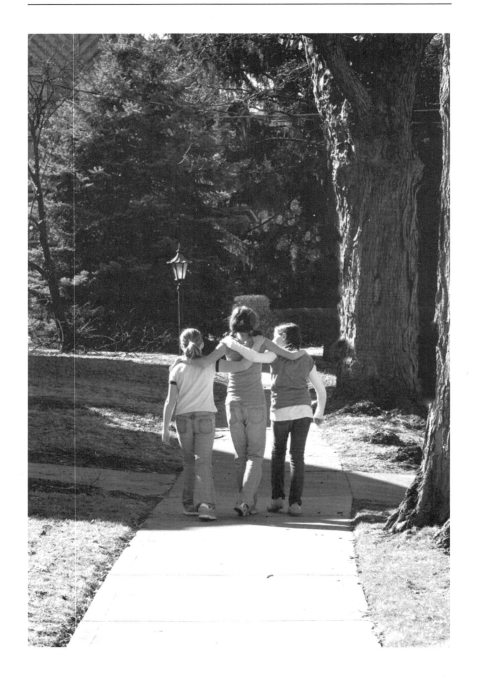

INTERVIEW QUESTIONNAIRE
Life Begins and Ends with Girlfriends
Ages 20-85+

When possible and appropriate, please indicate what age you were when an event took place.

1. How are your girlfriend (ships) different from other relationships in your life?

2. Describe times in your life when:

A. You have needed girlfriends and they were there.

B. You have needed girlfriends and they were not there.

3. Describe one or two events in your past when a girlfriend has played an important role. The role may have been positive or negative but days, or weeks, or years afterwards, you still remember.

4. Do you know women who do not have female friends?

Yes ☐

No ☐

Why do you suppose they do not have female friends?

5. Have your friendships with women changed over the course of your life?

Yes ☐

No ☐

Please describe.

6. Do you think that friendships among women **NOW** are different than they were for your mother or grandmother?

Yes ☐

No ☐

How and why?

7. At what points in your life have you been more eager to seek out female friends? How old were you at these times?

8. Have you consciously refrained from forming a girlfriend (ship) because you were afraid of the risks involved?

Yes   ☐

No   ☐

Can you describe what risks are involved in forming a girlfriend (ship)?

9. Friends often satisfy different needs in our lives. If that is true for you, please describe.

10. Are there some friendships that you keep even though you are not always able to be yourself with this person or persons?

Yes ☐

No ☐

Please describe.

11. Have you found it easier to confide in a girlfriend whom you don't know too well and/or may not see frequently?

Yes ☐

No ☐

Can you tell us why?

12. Think of a best girlfriend (past or current). How long has or was she your best girlfriend?

Explain how this person was involved in or has changed your life.

13. Have you ever had an experience that has shaken you to the core?

Yes ☐

No ☐

Did you tell a girlfriend?

Yes ☐

No ☐

Was her/their reaction expected or unexpected? Please explain.

14. Do your girlfriends substitute for family?

Yes ☐

No ☐

How and why?

15. What do you think that your girlfriend (ships) bring to your life that cannot or are not brought to you by family?

16. Please describe a time when you have been called upon to give preference to your family even though a good girlfriend needs or wants you to do something.

17. Have you been surprised in your life when you have faced something really difficult and the women you thought were your friends have disappointed you?

Yes ☐

No ☐

Who was left standing with you and why?

18. What is the best advice you could give to a young woman about the role and value of girlfriend (ships) in her life?

19. What lessons have you learned about girlfriend (ship) that you would want a young woman important to you to know? (Can be daughter, granddaughter, niece, sister, godchild, or other.)

20. Is there anything—a question, a topic, an issue—that we haven't mentioned that is important to you?

Please describe.

INTERVIEW QUESTIONNAIRE
Life Begins and Ends with Girlfriends
Ages 10–19

Thank you for completing this survey. We want to keep your answers private, so please do not write your name anywhere on this survey. When answering the following questions, think about your girl friend or girl friends (not your friends who are boys). Your answers will be kept strictly confidential.

1. Have there been times in your life when you really needed girl friends more than others?

    Yes ☐

    No ☐

    a. If yes, were your girl friends "there" for you during those times?

    Yes ☐

    No ☐

    b. If yes, describe one of those times when you needed a girl friend. What was going on?

c. If you answered no (that your girl friends were not "there" for you), what do you think was the reason?

2. Do you know a girl who does not have girl friends?

Yes ☐

No ☐

a. If yes, why do you think she does not have friends who are girls?

3. How old were you when you remember having your first "best" girl friend?

I was _____ years old.

a. Is she still your best friend?

Yes ☐

No ☐

i. If yes, how long has she been your "best friend"? _____

ii. If no, why is she no longer your best friend? What happened?

Do you have a new best girl friend?

Yes ☐

No ☐

4. Do you share "secrets" or private information with your girl friend or girl friends that you do not share with others?

☐ Yes ☐ No

5. Have you ever had to make a choice between doing something with your girl friend and spending time with your family?

Yes ☐

No ☐

a. If yes, did you choose spending time with your family or with your girl friend?

Family ☐

Friend ☐

   b. Why did you make the choice that you made?

6. What is the best advice you could give to another girl about having girl friends and making friends with other girls?

7. What lessons have you learned about your friendships with girls that you would want others to know?

Please tell us a little about yourself by filling in the blanks or circling your answer to the following questions.

1. I am _____ years old.

2. I am in the: 5th 6th 7th 8th 9th 10th 11th 12th grade

3. I have _____ brothers and _____ sisters.

4. I attend _____ public_____ private school.

5. I am: African-American_____
          White_____Hispanic_____ Asian_____
          Bi-racial_____   Other_____

About the Authors

Betsy Kyte Newman has been a professional educator all of her working life. The Cincinnati native grew up there, graduated from Manhattanville College, and returned to her hometown where she began her career as a high school English teacher and department head. She moved to San Francisco and University of California Berkeley to work on a doctorate and to teach at the university level. Marriage to businessman George Newman brought a cross-country move to Boston where their four children were born.

In Boston, Betsy continued university teaching and added consulting to the mix, founding her own firm there in 1982. She transferred her business to Cincinnati when the family returned in 1987.

Newman is a consultant in management education and career development, specializing in career planning, mid-career change, and life transitions. She conducts workshops and seminars on a national basis for prominent clients, including Merrill Lynch, Deloitte & Touche, Dow Jones/Wall Street Journal, and Procter & Gamble. Her previously published books are *Now That You've All Grown Up, What Do you Want to Be? (1996), Getting Unstuck: Moving Ahead With Your Career (2000)*, and *Retiring as a Career (2003)*.

Newman's now-adult children grew up in Cincinnati. They are a source of great pride, constant amazement—and endless, humbling learning. Two sons live in Cincinnati; one lawyer son is in Washington, D.C.; and her daughter is finishing law school in Cambridge.

Newman derives great joy from traveling and painting, and she loves books, movies, and the theater. She is an avid and enthusiastic artist, tennis player, walker, and occasional golfer.

Judy Van Ginkel lives and works in Cincinnati. She has a distinguished career as a champion for women's and children's health and has been honored by many groups including the Cincinnati Enquirer, Civic Ventures, Girl Scouts, Speaking of Women's Health, and the YWCA. Van Ginkel is Professor of Pediatrics at Cincinnati Children's Hospital and President of Every Child Succeeds (ECS), a large home-visitation program for first-time, at-risk mothers. The heart of ECS is the relationships that develop between the young mothers and the nurses/social workers who visit their homes—the quintessential girl friendships.

Judy is the mother of two girls and grandmother to two more. Her family is full of girls—sisters, cousins, stepdaughters, nieces. Her daughters both have successful careers but more importantly have good friends. The girls live away from Cincinnati where they grew up—Leigh Primack in Chicago and Jennifer Mooney in Florida.

When she was a small girl in Charleston, West Virginia, Van Ginkel went on house calls with her pediatrician father and finds it ironic that her life work now focuses on home visiting. Judy's mother stayed home, cared for her family, and volunteered in the community. Judy never saw herself with a career, although she always excelled in school and enjoyed learning. At 17, she went off alone to the University of Colorado. Within ten years of her college graduation, the world for women had changed. When her youngest daughter started first grade, Judy began her career by enrolling in a Ph.D. program at the University of Cincinnati.

When she isn't working, Judy enjoys exotic adventure travel with her husband, David, a pediatrician. They have been to most places in the world. The magpie part of her brings home baubles, beads, and gemstones that she transforms into jewelry—with the help of a skilled designer. She reads, walks, and misses her magnificent golden retrievers, Winston and Oliver, who died recently.

111

For Additional Copies of

Life Begins and Ends with

Girlfriends

Copy the form below or go to:
www.CincyBooks.com

Cincinnati Book Publishers
2449 Fairview Avenue
Cincinnati, OH 45219

PLEASE SEND ME _____ *COPIES*

MY CHECK FOR _____ IS ENCLOSED.
PLEASE MAKE CHECK PAYABLE TO: Cincinnati Book Publishers

1-5 COPIES $19.95 + $1.30 TAX* + $3 25 S&H = $24.50 EA. *Ohio residents
6-19 COPIES $17.95 + $1.17 TAX* + $2.38 S&H = 21.50 EA.   only
20+ COPIES $15.95 + $1.04 TAX* + 2.01 S&H = 19.00 EA.

NAME

ADDRESS

CITY   STATE   ZIP

PHONE   EMAIL

VISA   MASTERCARD   DISCOVER   AMERICAN EXPRESS
(CIRCLE ONE)

CARD #   EX DATE

NAME ON CARD

THANK YOU!

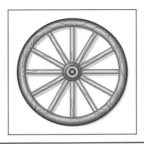

THE TRAVELER'S GUIDE TO
THE OREGON TRAIL

by
Julie Fanselow

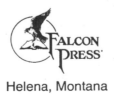

FALCON PRESS

Helena, Montana

For Bruce,
my partner in life's travels

Library of Congress Catalog Card Number: 92-055085

ISBN: 1-56044-192-5

Falcon Press Publishing Co., Inc.
P.O. Box 1718, Helena, MT 59624

♻ Text pages printed on recycled paper.

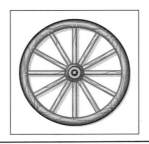

ACKNOWLEDGMENTS

Many people contributed to the creation of this book. I must first thank the people at Wild Horse Studio here in Twin Falls, Idaho, who hired me to write copy for an Oregon Trail map covering our state. It was that project that convinced me of the need for a modern travel guide to the trail.

A number of people offered advice and suggestions to me during my research and travels. The staff of each state's travel and tourism department showered me with invaluable information. Especially helpful were Mary Ethel Emanuel of the Nebraska Division of Travel and Tourism; Linda Sauer of the Wyoming Division of Tourism; Georgia Smith of the Idaho Department of Commerce; the staff of Nebraska's I-80 rest areas; and the staff of the National Oregon Trail Interpretive Center in Baker City, Oregon.

Many other authors have written about the Oregon Trail, but I owe a particular debt of gratitude to Gregory Franzwa, owner of the Patrice Press. His *The Oregon Trail Revisited* and *Maps of the Oregon Trail* were invaluable references, and I turned to them countless times while researching and writing this book.

Others deserving·thanks include Julia Anderson and Bill Kelley of Vancouver, Washington, who provided a good night's rest and timely truck cap repairs near the end of the Oregon Trail; my neighbor, Helen Anderson, whose copy of *Maps of the Oregon Trail* proved my best friend along the trail; my sister-in-law, Kay Phillips, and nieces Risa, Jami and Bree, who gave me a great tour of Fort Caspar; and Andy Arenz of The Times-News for photographic assistance at the 1992 Three Island Crossing re-enactment.

Thanks also go to the Swetye family, with whom I made my first trips West, and to the people at Falcon Press, especially Mac Bates, Will Harmon, and Randall Green.

Finally, thanks to the three most important people in my life: my father, Byron Fanselow, who taught me a love of history and of learning; my brother, Jeff Fanselow, who knows the value of adventure and an inquiring mind; and my best friend and husband, Bruce Whiting, who always encourages me to follow my path wherever it might lead.

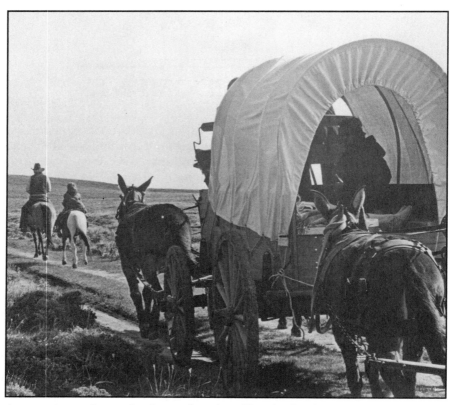

A re-enactment shows what it must have been like traveling by wagon train along the Oregon Trail in the 1800s. Photo courtesy of Wyoming Division of Tourism.

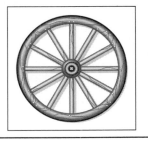

FOREWORD

Lured by tales of land, gold, and a new life, more than 300,000 Americans migrated westward on the Oregon Trail system during the mid-nineteenth century. Stretching from Independence, Missouri, to the Willamette River Valley in Oregon, the primitive route promised—and delivered—a difficult journey. Emigrants battled unforgiving terrain, extreme weather, poor equipment, illness, and occasional attacks from Indians, who viewed the wagon trains with increasingly wary eyes. But the travelers pressed on across the plains and mountains, ready to endure the Wild West's risks and rigors, eager to see and settle in Oregon's lush river valleys or find their fortunes in golden California.

The year 1993 marks the sesquicentennial—or 150th anniversary—of the first wagon train's arrival at the Oregon Trail's end. Many good books have been written about the trail and can guide the modern visitor to the exact routes the pioneers traveled, mile by mile across the continent. But few, if any, books have provided today's traveler with a guide both to the trail's history and present-day attractions nearby. That is what this book aims to do. Whether you have a long weekend, a two-week vacation, or just a favorite armchair, you can use this guide to help you get a taste of the Oregon Trail.

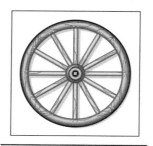

CONTENTS

THE OREGON TRAIL

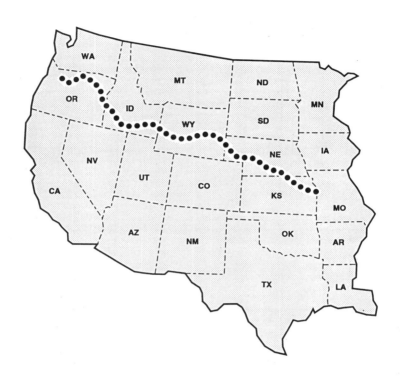

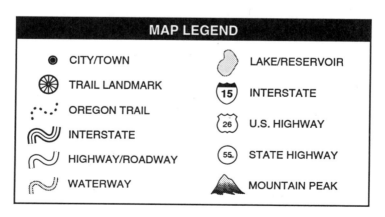

MAP LEGEND	
◉ CITY/TOWN	🗇 LAKE/RESERVOIR
⊕ TRAIL LANDMARK	15 INTERSTATE
⋯⋅⋅⋅ OREGON TRAIL	26 U.S. HIGHWAY
∿ INTERSTATE	55 STATE HIGHWAY
∿ HIGHWAY/ROADWAY	🗻 MOUNTAIN PEAK
∿ WATERWAY	

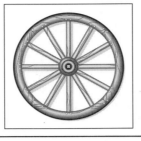

CHAPTER ONE

THE OREGON TRAIL: A BRIEF HISTORY AND OVERVIEW

To many, the idea seemed preposterous. Why would anyone want to leave the safety of the United States to push into unknown country? Why would anyone willingly choose to endure six months of choking dust, searing heat, and rain-swollen river crossings along a trail lined with grave sites and discarded possessions?

The pioneers had their reasons. Many were fed up with poor Eastern soil, which had become overpriced, overcrowded, and worn thin through excessive cultivation. Land in the Oregon country, by contrast, was plentiful and dirt cheap. And what a land it was rumored to be! Why, in Oregon, beets were said to grow three feet in diameter and turnips five feet around. One trail proponent even told would-be emigrants that, in Oregon, "the pigs are running about under the great acorn trees, round and fat, and already cooked, with knives and forks sticking in them so that you can cut off a slice whenever you are hungry." Who could resist such tales of plenty, even if they were somewhat, ah, exaggerated?

Other emigrants were motivated by pure patriotism and the notion of "manifest destiny." In the early nineteenth century, the Northwest was still shared with the British, but many emigrants felt sure that if enough Americans settled in Oregon, the United States could lay a legitimate sole claim to the area. It worked, too; Oregon was awarded territorial status in 1849 and became a state just one decade later, thirty-one years before either neighboring Idaho or Washington attained statehood.

Finally, many pioneers simply had the urge to push ever westward as their ancestors had done for generations—from Europe to the New

World, from Plymouth Rock to Philadelphia, from Pennsylvania across the Alleghenies to Ohio and Kentucky and Missouri and on across the plains. This trip would not disappoint them, for although it was long and potentially dangerous, it boasted the most amazing scenery they had ever viewed. Wide-horizoned plains gave way to jagged mountains and steep canyons, then fragrant pine forests. And at the end, Oregon, promising land enough for everybody and a new start on life.

By the time the first emigrant wagon trains rolled in the 1840s, the Oregon Trail was a well-known route. Native Americans had long ago pioneered the way. Lewis and Clark sparked white settlers' interest in the West after President Thomas Jefferson dispatched their Corps of Discovery to survey the lands acquired in the Louisiana Purchase. Inspired by Lewis and Clark, New York fur dealer John Jacob Astor sent parties to build trading posts along the Columbia River.

The Astorians, as they came to be known, were the first whites to discover the South Pass route through the Rockies. Later, brave mountain men set off to discover firsthand the beaver and buffalo, the mountains and raging rivers, and the curious, self-assured Native Americans.

The real push took place, however, after missionaries Marcus Whitman and Samuel Parker traveled from Liberty, Missouri, to the West in 1835. Convinced by the efforts of earlier missionaries such as Jason Lee that Indians wanted the white man's "medicine"—Christianity—Whitman returned the next year to establish a mission on the Walla Walla River. The trip made history for two reasons. First, Whitman brought along his brand new wife, Narcissa Prentiss Whitman, who— along with Eliza Spalding, wife of missionary Henry Spalding—would become the first white woman to travel the road to Oregon. Together, they proved families could make the trip. Second, the Whitmans traveled by wagon, and although their vehicle didn't last the entire journey, they showed wheeled passage was possible. The missionaries succeeded in establishing the first white settlements in the Pacific Northwest, and by 1840, at least 100 men, women, and children had arrived from the United States.

After that, the tide of emigration swelled. Stories appeared in the national press and exciting letters streamed in from neighbors who had made the journey. In 1843, about 1,000 people left Independence for Oregon. Two years later, more than 3,000 people made the trip, and in 1847, as many as 4,000 folks signed on. But busiest of all were the gold rush years of 1849 through 1852, when tens of thousands of people followed the overland route as far as present-day Idaho before cutting southwest to California.

A typical trip along the 2,000-mile trail took about five months, with emigrants traveling at the rate of just fifteen to twenty hard, dusty miles per day. The journey usually started late in April or early in May, as soon as the grass had grown high enough to feed the livestock that would be making the trip.

In the trail's early days, Independence was the main supply post and jumping-off spot. Emigrants often arrived at Independence by steamboat from St. Louis and points east. Once there, they'd organize into wagon trains and make final preparations for the journey.

Most important was the wagon, which most emigrants already had obtained by the time they arrived on the frontier. In his guidebook *The Prairie Traveler: A Handbook for Overland Expedition*, Captain R.B. Marcy said wagons should be simple, strong, and light, made of well-seasoned timber. He recommended that wheels be made of osage orange or white oak to prevent shrinkage in the hot, dry West. The wagon bed—frequently built by the emigrant himself—was ten to eleven feet long, four feet wide, and two feet deep. A good wagon cost about $85.

Emigrants often argued over whether to use mules or oxen for the trip. Many favored mules because, with good roads and plenty of grain, they could travel fast and stand up to the heat. But a six-mule team cost $600. Oxen, on the other hand, cost just $200 for eight and had more stamina over the long run. Oxen also were less likely to stampede and could be used for food. In addition to the mules or oxen, most parties brought along a few cows for milk.

After the wagon and stock were obtained, the emigrants set about filling it with their provisions. The following grocery list was typical for a family of four: 824 pounds of flour, 725 pounds of bacon, seventy-five pounds of coffee, 160 pounds of sugar, 200 pounds of lard and suet, 200 pounds of beans, 135 pounds of peaches and apples, and salt, pepper, and bicarbonate of soda.

Once on the road, the emigrants started each day before dawn, awakened by a trumpet reverie or a gunshot blast at 4 a.m. They'd usually hit the trail within a couple of hours, eager to start the day's journey so they could be that much closer to Oregon. Emigrants rarely rode in the wagons, for the vehicles were small, full of possessions, and hardly comfortable for traveling. Instead, they walked alongside. The trains traveled all day except for an hour "nooning" break at midday.

Finally, at about 6 p.m., the pioneers would draw their wagons into a circle to ward off intruders and form a corral for the stock. Everyone would wander off to collect buffalo chips for the evening fire. After dinner, the emigrants would often enjoy singing, dancing, and storytelling around the crackling campfire.

The Oregon Trail has sometimes been described as "the world's longest graveyard." Cholera killed thousands. Others died by accidental gunshot or rattlesnake bite. Indian attacks claimed a few lives. In all, about one in seventeen adults died along the trail. For kids, the toll was even higher. Of every five children who started the trip, one would fail to finish. Emigrants who died were often buried right on the trail, where wagon wheels rolling over the fresh plot would help hide the body from coyotes, wolves, and grave-robbers.

Although a mile of trail could contain as many as fifteen graves, most who started the trip survived to see Oregon and tell tales of the great adventure for many years to come. By the time Oregon Trail travel trickled off in the mid-1860s, more than 300,000 people had moved to the West Coast. Propelled by patriotism, driven by a restless spirit, Americans had made the greatest peacetime migration in the history of the world. The frontier was closed. "Manifest destiny" was secure, for better or for worse. The United States was truly one nation, indivisible, from sea to shining sea.

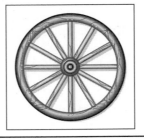

CHAPTER TWO

HOW TO USE THIS BOOK

To follow every twist and turn in the primary route of the Oregon Trail would take about a month. There are guidebooks to help the reader do just that—most notably Gregory M. Franzwa's *The Oregon Trail Revisited* and an excellent, spiral-bound atlas, *Maps of the Oregon Trail*, by the same author. But *The Traveler's Guide to the Oregon Trail* assumes a different type of trail traveler.

You are fascinated with the Oregon Trail, its tales of human drama and its meaning in American history, and you'd like to see many of the trail's highlights. But like most people, your vacation time is limited. And you have other interests in addition to exploring history: hiking, camping, fishing, swimming, rodeo, golf, rock climbing, rafting, or just plain sightseeing and relaxing.

This guidebook provides information on all the major Oregon Trail historic sites as well as places to eat, sleep, and play along the trail of today. The next section of this chapter presents a nine-day trip (suited to those with two-week vacations). This nine-day trip gives a good overview of what life was like along the Oregon Trail. Those who can't spare nine days this trip can always do half the trail this year and half some other time. Or split the trail into three long weekends. The most important thing is to adjust the trip to your own interests, learning about the trail while savoring your favorite leisure activities. We want you to arrive home feeling as if you've had a vacation, after all!

SUGGESTED TRIP

The following is a suggested nine-day trip along the Oregon Trail. Approximate driving times and distances are given, along with major stops en route. More specific instructions to places listed are given in the appropriate later chapters. Please remember this trip plan is only a suggestion and can easily be modified to suit your family's interests and needs.

Day One: From St. Louis to Independence, Missouri—Start in St. Louis by visiting the **Gateway Arch and Museum of Westward Expansion**. After lunch, drive west on Interstate 70 to **Arrow Rock, Missouri**, where a state historic site and several private businesses preserve what was once an important stop for many settlers on their way to the frontier. Drive on to Independence for the evening.
Approximate driving time/distance: five hours, 275 miles

Day Two: From Independence, Missouri, to Manhattan, Kansas—Begin the day with a visit to the **National Frontier Trails Center** in Independence. Drive on into Kansas City to visit **Westport**, a district where emigrants made final preparations for the trip west. After lunch in Kansas City, take I-70 to U.S. Highway 75 at Topeka. Follow U.S. 75 north two miles to U.S. Route 24. Afternoon stops along or near Route 24 should include **St. Marys Mission** at the town of St. Marys, which was an Oregon Trail resting stop, and the **Vermillion River Crossing** near Louisville. Overnight at Manhattan, Kansas.
Approximate driving time/distance: three hours, 180 miles

Day Three: From Manhattan, Kansas, to Kearney, Nebraska—Leave Manhattan via Route 24 and drive northwest to U.S. Route 77. This morning, visit **Alcove Spring** near Blue Rapids. (Permission must be obtained before entering; see the Kansas chapter for details.) Continue on Route 77 to Marysville, turn left (west) on U.S. Highway 36, then watch for the signs at State Route 148 for the **Hollenberg Ranch**, a favorite Oregon Trail campsite and Pony Express station. In the afternoon, visit **Rock Creek Station State Historical Park** near Fairbury, Nebraska, then drive on via Routes 136, 81, and 6 to Minden, home of Harold Warp's Pioneer Village. End the day with a visit to **Fort Kearny State Park,** and spend the night at Kearney.
Approximate driving time/distance: 5.5 hours, 250 miles

Day Four: From Kearney, Nebraska, to Scottsbluff, Nebraska—Today's itinerary includes some of the most famous sights along the Oregon Trail. Take Interstate 80 west from Kearney to Ogallala, stopping en route if time permits to see **Midway Station** south of Gothenburg and **O'Fallon's Bluff** near Sutherland. Exit at Ogallala and take U.S.

Highway 30 west to Brule to visit the excellent trail ruts at **California Hill**. Proceed on U.S. Highway 26 to **Ash Hollow State Historical Park**, making sure to stop first to see the steep and dangerous descent wagons faced at **Windlass Hill**. Continue west on Highway 26 to see **Courthouse and Jail rocks** near Bridgeport and **Chimney Rock** near Bayard. Spend the night at Scottsbluff.

Approximate driving time/distance: five hours, 275 miles (Time zone change from Central to Mountain)

Day Five: From Scottsbluff, Nebraska, to Casper, Wyoming— Before leaving Nebraska, drive to the top of **Scotts Bluff National Monument**, another major trail landmark. The first stop in Wyoming will be **Fort Laramie**, a center of activity for pioneers, military personnel, Indians, and fur traders. Next, visit Guernsey, where emigrants signed their names on **Register Cliff** and left some of the deepest wagon-wheel ruts remaining anywhere along the Oregon Trail. Pick up Interstate 25 about fifteen miles west of Guernsey and drive to **Ayres Natural Bridge** near Douglas. From there, continue on I-25 to Casper, where **Fort Caspar** marks a crossing of the North Platte River. Spend the night in Casper.

Approximate driving time/distance: three hours, 175 miles

Day Six: From Casper, Wyoming, to Kemmerer, Wyoming— (Special note: hit the road early for this longest day on the trail. If an extra day is available, split this itinerary in half, overnighting in Lander.) Drive southwest of Casper on State Route 220. Make a brief stop at Bessemer Bend to see the **Red Buttes**, noted in many emigrant diaries. Drive on to **Independence Rock**, where pioneers often spent the Fourth of July. **Devil's Gate**, another landmark, is just a few miles west. Take U.S. Highway 287 heading northwest at Muddy Gap Junction and drive to the intersection with State Route 28 south of Lander. Follow Route 28 south and watch for the signs to South Pass City, a restored historical mining town. (The actual South Pass crossing of the Continental Divide is nearby; see the Wyoming chapter for directions.) Take Route 28 and U.S. Highway 191 south to Rock Springs, then travel west on Interstate 80 to **Fort Bridger**, established by the famous mountain man Jim Bridger as an outfitting post. From Fort Bridger, take Wyoming Route 412 or U.S. Highway 189 north to Kemmerer, where travelers can spend the night before heading into Idaho.

Approximate driving time/distance: seven hours, 380 miles

Day Seven: From Kemmerer, Wyoming, to Twin Falls, Idaho— Take U.S. Highway 30 into Idaho. The day's first stop will be at **Soda Springs**, where emigrants marveled at one spring with water that tasted like beer and another that sounded like a steamboat. At the junction of Interstate 15, head north to Pocatello and visit the replica of **Fort Hall.**

Turn west on Interstate 86 and drive to **Massacre Rocks State Park,** surrounded by the lava fields that characterize this part of Idaho. Continue on Interstate 86 and Interstate 84 to Burley, where Route 30 comes in. The **Milner Ruts** Bureau of Land Management Interpretive Area boasts some fine wagon ruts. Approaching Twin Falls, visit the **Stricker Store,** where emigrants often camped, and **Shoshone Falls,** which many pioneers heard but never saw. Overnight in Twin Falls.

Approximate driving time/distance: five hours, 280 miles

Day Eight: From Twin Falls, Idaho, to Baker City, Oregon— Leave Twin Falls on Route 30, which leads through the Hagerman Valley, where emigrants saw water cascading from the Snake River Canyon wall at **Thousand Springs.** Return to Interstate 84 at Bliss and drive west to Glenns Ferry, site of the **Three Island Crossing,** one of the trail's most difficult river fords. **Bonneville Point,** located near Exit 64, was where travelers first saw the green Boise River Valley that marked the desert's end. Parma is home to a replica of the Hudson's Bay Company's **Fort Boise.** Once in Oregon, Interstate 84 parallels the trail past **Farewell Bend** and the **Burnt River Canyon.** Take Exit 302 (Oregon Route 86) at Baker City to **Flagstaff Hill,** home of the BLM's Oregon Trail Interpretive Center. Visit the center and spend the night in Baker City.

Approximate driving time/distance: 4.5 hours, 250 miles (Time zone change from Mountain to Pacific)

Day Nine: From Baker City, Oregon, to Oregon City, Oregon— Drive through the Grande Ronde Valley and into the Blue Mountains, stopping at Emigrant Springs State Park near the summit. (At Pendleton, consider a sidetrip north to Walla Walla, Washington, site of the Whitman Mission.) Continue west on I-84 to **The Dalles.** Here, the emigrants had to make a choice and today's travelers will, too: Either continue on down the **Columbia River** (stay on Interstate 84) or take the overland **Barlow Road** south of Mount Hood. Whichever way is choosen, trail's end is reached at **Oregon City,** on I-205 southeast of Portland.

Approximate driving time/distance: 5.5 hours, 320 miles (via I-84 instead of the Barlow Road)

Some people won't have time to see the entire trail. If you have only a few days to travel, or if you would like to work a short Oregon Trail sojourn into your vacation elsewhere out West, consider the following: Get off Interstate 80 at Ogallala, Nebraska, and follow this book from there to Guernsey, Wyoming. This 190-mile stretch offers many of the best, most scenic, and most historic Oregon Trail landmarks, including California Hill, Windlass Hill, Ash Hollow, Courthouse Rock, Chimney

Rock, Scotts Bluff, Fort Laramie, and the outstanding trail ruts at Guernsey. The terrain is classic American West: broad horizons, strange and beautiful rock formations, miles and miles without a town. What's more, this trip doesn't range too far afield; travelers can hop on I-25 just fifteen miles west of Guernsey and get back on I-80 at Cheyenne a mere hour-and-a-half later.

WHEN TO GO

The emigrants started their journey by mid-spring, aiming to reach Oregon's Blue Mountains before the snow flew in October or November. Today's pioneers should make the trip sometime during the same seasons to best see what the pioneers saw.

June may be the best month to make the journey. Go earlier, and suffer chilly nights, spring rains, and impassable roads; wait until later in the summer, and endure oppressive heat crossing the high, arid stretches of trail through Wyoming, Idaho, and eastern Oregon, where temperatures regularly push the 100-degree mark in July and August.

Western weather is unpredictable and sometimes extreme. High winds and sudden heavy rains can occur any time during the spring, summer, and fall. But don't worry if the weather turns nasty—there are excellent museums and plenty of other indoor diversions along the trail route where travelers can pass time until the clouds blow past (or the heat dies down).

HOW TO TRAVEL

Most people will want to start their Oregon Trail trek from either St. Louis or Independence, Missouri, both located on Interstate 70. Although it will add a day to the trip, a start in St. Louis works best for several reasons. First, the city served as a funnel for the pioneers, with many boarding steamboats here for the trip up the Missouri River to Independence and the actual jumping-off points for Oregon. Second, St. Louis is home to the Gateway Arch and Museum of Westward Expansion, which does a great job of interpreting not just the pioneer trails but the whole history of Americans pushing west.

Situated as it is in middle America, Missouri is within two to three long days of driving for anyone in the continental United States. Here's an extreme case: with only two weeks—actually sixteen days, with weekends—for vacation, a determined sightseer could drive from Boston or Miami to St. Louis (about 1,200 miles, either way) in two days, take the suggested nine-day trip to Oregon City, and still be home (after another five-day haul back across the country) in time to return to work. But if time is limited or home is really far from the trailhead, then fly to St. Louis or Kansas City, rent a vehicle, drive to Oregon, and fly home from Portland.

The Oregon-bound pioneers rarely blazed new trails. Most of the route had been used for centuries, first by Native Americans, later by explorers, trappers, and mountain men. These guys knew what they were doing, and the routes they picked—mostly by following rivers—still are used today.

Because much of the Oregon Trail runs either beneath or within several miles of our modern-day highways, any family car in good condition should be able to make the trip without trouble. This book describes several side trips off the beaten path, and these too can all be traversed in a typical two-wheel-drive vehicle. (My pickup truck, with minimal clearance, more than 100,000 miles, and a measly four cylinders, was subjected to all routes described and survived intact.)

To get way off the beaten path, take a four-wheel-drive vehicle. Anyone hoping to follow Gregory Franzwa's detailed route mile by mile would need a four-by-four, as would anyone who wanted to make the trip in early spring, since even the "easy" back roads can prove muddy in April and May.

Air conditioning serves two purposes in Oregon Trail country: climate control and dust abatement. For those traveling with air conditioning, make sure to get out of the vehicle often enough to actually feel the hot, dry air and the dust, both constant companions to the westering emigrants. Those without air conditioning can console themselves with the knowledge that the pioneers didn't have it, either, and today's "covered wagons" make a heck of a lot better time than the prairie schooners did. At any rate, it's wise to wear light-colored, airy clothes and drink plenty of fluids.

Air conditioning may be a luxury, but don't forego any of the following: dashboard compass, working odometer, full-size spare tire and jack, gasoline can, shovel (in case the trail's mud claims yet another set of wheels), and some kind of basic emergency kit including flashers. The truth is, although most of the trail follows modern roads, many black-topped Western highways are as lonesome as the most desolate back road in the East or Midwest. Make sure your car or truck is in good shape before starting out, paying particular attention to tires, belts, and hoses. And once on the road, keep an eye on the gas gauge—it's fifty miles or more between filling stations in some areas.

A word about side trips: out West, distances between towns are so much greater that most natives are accustomed to driving vast stretches without thinking much of it. Whereas Easterners may pale at the thought of driving from Pittsburgh to Chicago—a distance of 475 miles, many Westerners regularly cover as many miles just to shop at a larger town. And some folks out West can travel 475 miles in one direction without crossing a state line!

Of course, some travelers quickly adapt to this new scale. My first time out West, my companion and I were huddled one rainy morning in a soggy tent in Rocky Mountain National Park. It dawned on us that Arches National Park, where rain was unlikely, was a mere six- or seven-hour drive away. So we went, of course. We camped that night south of Moab, Utah, in time to see an incredible moonrise in the clear, starry night air.

Bear this in mind when a side trip beckons to Yellowstone National Park, Oregon's Wallowa Mountains, or the Badlands of South Dakota. Reckon the additional distances—and days needed—carefully. Weigh this against your need to change scenery, or to escape bad weather or crowds. For those who do decide to stray, this book includes information on many famous Western destinations—most within 150 miles of the Oregon Trail.

Finally, just a few rules for traveling in the West. Most of the areas described in this book are open to the public, but a few require permission to enter. If that is the case, please respect the landowner's wishes and consult with the property owner before proceeding. If access is uncertain, the nearest Bureau of Land Management or Forest Service office is often the best place to find out who owns the land in question. Whether on private or public land, treat it with care. Close any gate that you open, stay on the main trails, and refrain from littering or otherwise spoiling the view for others.

WHERE TO STAY; WHAT TO EAT

Each of the following chapters ends with a list of lodging options, campgrounds, and restaurants for each area along the trail. The listings follow the Oregon Trail from east to west. In most cases, establishments mentioned are simply representative of what is available in each town; listing in this guidebook does not imply endorsement of any kind.

Many modern-day pioneers will want to camp at least part of the way. Sleeping outdoors gives a better taste of what pioneer life was like, and it helps save money, too. My favored routine of cross-country travel calls for camping out in a tent two to three nights in a row, followed by one night in a motel or staying with friends en route. I'm convinced one of life's greatest pleasures is a long, hot shower and nice, soft bed after a few days of "roughing it."

State park facilities are often the best bet along the route. Aside from being plentiful, state park campgrounds usually offer clean and scenic grounds, shower facilities, friendly advice, and easy access. Most are quite reasonable, too, charging from $4 to $10 per night (although many state parks now charge vehicle admission fees which can add a few dollars to the tab).

Because the Oregon Trail follows so many major highways, motels are plentiful. And because so much of the route is far from urban America, rates are quite reasonable. The national budget chains are well represented, but even better deals are sometimes found at independent "mom-and-pop" motels tucked away from the interstate in nearly every town. Some AAA-listed motels run as low as $20-25 for two people. Hotel, motel, and bed-and-breakfast rates listed in this guidebook are generally for double occupancy during the summer travel season and were accurate as of 1992.

Driving and sightseeing take up a lot of time on an Oregon Trail trip, so quick-and-simple meals are best. Restaurants are plentiful in most regions, but economical lunches and snacks can be carried in a well-stocked cooler.

The restaurants listed in these pages disclose my bias toward locally owned eateries. Many offer regional specialties and down-home cooking unavailable at the national chains, and prices are often in line with those at fast-food joints. Nevertheless, most good-sized towns along the interstate highways will have several chain restaurants in addition to the locally owned spots.

More complete lists of hotels, motels, campgrounds, and restaurants are available from state and local tourism bureaus, many of which have toll-free phone numbers for information. State tourism offices are listed at the end of this chapter, and local offices are listed throughout the book.

WHAT TO PACK

If you're camping with kids and they are old enough, pack along two tents. Most kids love to have a tent of their own, and having separate tents will give the grown-ups some privacy and quiet, too, always prized on a long road trip. As mentioned earlier, skies along the trail can be unpredictable, so make sure the tent is waterproof, pack along a ground cloth, and put up the fly. Wind is another constant on the plains, so remember the tent stakes, too.

Other camp essentials include a simple tool kit with a hammer, axe, and pocket knife; a reliable camp stove and fuel (especially since campfires are prohibited in some locations); cooking and eating utensils; a can opener; insect repellent; a water bucket for hauling water and washing dishes; biodegradable dish soap; rope (for clothesline or other uses); first-aid and snake-bite kits; a camp lantern and flashlights; matches; trash bags; and a bag for dirty laundry.

Starting an Oregon Trail trip with a flight to Missouri doesn't mean camping is out of the question. Some state parks and campgrounds offer either cabins or rent-a-camp sites, and a few are equipped with all the essential gear. One note of caution: many rental cabins, while slightly cheaper than most motel rooms, offer no motel-type amenities other than a roof over your head. Bring a sleeping bag and cooking and eating utensils...even a lantern.

As for clothing, it's best to be prepared. In summer, bring plenty of short-sleeved shirts and shorts. But toss in long pants, sweaters, and a jacket, too, because early mornings and nights can be chilly. Sneakers will suffice for walks around many historic sites, but most travelers will want a pair of hiking boots, too.

Still have room? Toss in a swimsuit and sun block. Remember a camera, and a wide-angle lens for those high, wide horizons. Binoculars might come in handy, as will books and travel games. Finally, don't forget maps—the ones in this book are general and should always be used in conjunction with a more detailed local highway map.

TRAVELING WITH KIDS

A trip along the Oregon Trail makes an ideal family vacation. It's interesting, educational, informal, and can easily be blended in with a more traditional Western vacation to the national parks and landmarks. Best of all, it is blessedly easy on the pocketbook, since most historic sites are free or cheap, and since most of the trail winds far from expensive cities and theme parks.

Still, kids will be kids, and looking for ways to keep them happy and occupied is always a challenge. Throughout the book, I've made note of free or low-cost recreational activities that can give children a chance to blow off a little steam—playgrounds, parks, and pools are especially good. Some historic sites offer programs just for kids, and these are mentioned, too.

One activity that can be planned in advance is an Oregon Trail scavenger hunt. Before the trip, make a list of things the kids can look for along the way. The list might include such items as a covered wagon, Chimney Rock, Indian tipi, pronghorn antelope, Pony Express station, cactus, sod house, wagon ruts, deer, Independence Rock, fort, and river. For extra fun, give the kids an inexpensive camera so they can take photos of the discoveries as they are made.

Kids love to have a little bit of their own money to spend on vacation, and this helps teach them financial responsibility and decision making. Consider giving each child a special trip allowance. Make sure they know that this allowance should cover any souvenirs they want to buy and it must last the whole trip.

WHAT TO READ

Many travelers want to read more about the Oregon Trail before, during, or after following the route. Especially recommended, in addition to the Franzwa books already mentioned, are the following volumes:

Historic Sites Along the Oregon Trail by Aubrey L. Haines; *The Way West*, a novel by A.B. Guthrie Jr.; *The Wake of the Prairie Schooner* by Irene D. Paden, who spent many years tracing the trails with her family; and *Along the Oregon Trail*, a series of newspaper columns written by Missouri journalist Donna Reinheimer McGuire, who traveled the route in 1988.

Trail buffs also may want to consider a membership in the Oregon-California Trails Association, which helps mark, interpret, and preserve the trails. Members receive *Overland Journal* and *News From the Plains* and can take part in local chapter activities. For information, write OCTA at P.O. Box 1019, Independence, MO 64051-2276.

STATE TOURISM OFFICES

Missouri Division of Tourism

Truman Office Building, P.O. Box 1055, Jefferson City, MO 65102

(314) 751-4133

Kansas Travel & Tourism Division

700 S.W. Harrison, Suite 1200, Topeka, KS 66603

(913) 296-2009

Nebraska Travel & Tourism Division

P.O. Box 94666, 700 S. 16th, Lincoln, NE 68509

(800) 228-4307 or (402) 471-3800

Wyoming Division of Tourism

I-25 at College Drive, Cheyenne, WY 82002

(800) 225-5996 or (307) 777-7777

Idaho Division of Tourism Development

700 W. State St., Boise, ID 83720

(800) 635-7820 or (208) 334-2470

Oregon Tourism Division

775 Summer St. N.E., Salem, OR 97310

(800) 547-7842

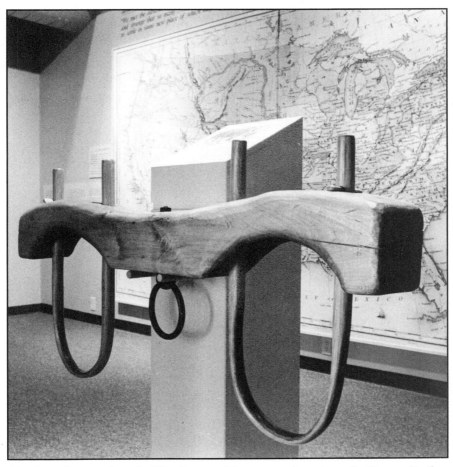

Wooden oxbows and a yoke like those used by many emigrants on the Oregon Trail are on display at the National Frontier Trails Center in Independence, Missouri. Photo courtesy of the Missouri Division of Tourism.

IS THIS BOOK OUT OF DATE?

As this book was being researched and written, communities all along the Oregon Trail were in the midst of planning their celebrations of the trail's 150th anniversary. Several towns expect to open brand-new interpretive centers; others may expand or change the facilities already in place.

Of course, other things may change, too. Restaurants and motels may change names, and visitor attractions mentioned in these pages may alter operating schedules.

If you spot an error, omission, or change, please write me in care of Falcon Press, P.O. Box 1718, Helena, MT 59624. We will use your input in future editions of *The Traveler's Guide to the Oregon Trail.* May you have many happy travels!

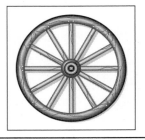

CHAPTER THREE

BOLD BEGINNINGS: MISSOURI AND KANSAS

"A multitude of shops had sprung up to furnish the emigrants and Santa Fe travelers with necessaries for their long journey and there was an incessant hammering and banging from a dozen blacksmiths' sheds, where the heavy wagons were being repaired, and the horses and oxen shod."
—Francis Parkman at Independence Square, 1846

ST. LOUIS, MISSOURI, AND THE GATEWAY ARCH

They came, mostly from Arkansas, Missouri, Kentucky, and Illinois. For months they'd discussed going west to Oregon, and now the time had arrived. Wide-eyed with excitement, they arrived in St. Louis ready to begin the adventure of their lifetimes.

St. Louis has long been known as "Gateway to the West." Today, most people would argue that the West really begins some 500 miles west of St. Louis, where the 100th Meridian streaks past the likes of Dodge City, Kansas. But St. Louis is where the idea of westward expansion began both in theory and in practice. Nowhere is this better explained than at the **Jefferson National Expansion Memorial** and its centerpiece, the **Gateway Arch.**

One of the nation's greatest monuments, the Gateway Arch is also the tallest at 630 feet. (The Washington Monument, by contrast, is 555

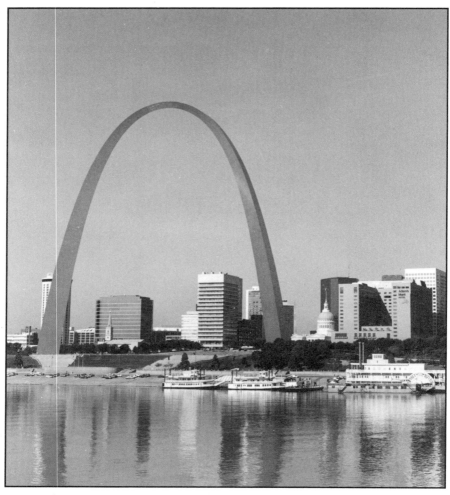

*The 630-foot-tall Gateway Arch towers above the city of St. Louis, Missouri.
Photo courtesy of the Missouri Division of Tourism.*

feet tall and the Statue of Liberty reaches a mere 305 feet into the sky.) Finnish-American architect Eero Saarinen's design for the stainless steel rainbow won a national contest in 1947; unfortunately, he died in 1961, a year before the Arch's construction actually began. The monument was completed in October 1965, and more than fifty million people have visited since its opening.

A ride to the top of the Arch is a thrilling experience. After a four-minute trip up the Arch's innards in a space-capsule-like tram car, visitors reach an observation room with vistas thirty miles both east and west on a clear day. Some of the best sights, however, are spread at the Arch's feet—the Mississippi River and its fancy riverboats, Busch Stadium and the Old Courthouse, the green jewel of the parkland around the Arch, and the bright blue swimming pools atop downtown hotels.

During peak visitation seasons, a tram leaves for the top every five minutes from 8:30 a.m. to 9:10 p.m. Despite these frequent departures, there may be a short wait. During the off-season, rides are offered every 10 to 20 minutes from 9:30 a.m. to 5:10 p.m. Tickets cost $2.50 for anyone 13 or older and fifty cents for children ages three through twelve.

To learn more about the Arch and how it was built, see "Monument to the Dream," a thirty-five-minute film shown in the Tucker Theater beneath the Arch. The film is shown every forty-five minutes and admission is $1 per person. Another theater opened in 1992 featuring showings of such Ultra 70mm large-format films as "To Fly" and "Secrets of the Grand Canyon."

The Museum of Westward Expansion also sits beneath the Arch. In its center is a life-size statue of Thomas Jefferson, who presided over the Louisiana Purchase and sent Meriwether Lewis and William Clark forth from Missouri to survey the new lands. From the statue, museum displays radiate outward in semi-circles, each describing a key aspect of westward movement between 1803—the date of the Louisiana Purchase—and 1890, when the frontier was officially declared closed.

National Park Service rangers lead guided tours through the museum every hour. Visitors can also wander through on their own. Displays include an overland wagon, a pioneer sod house, and exhibits on mountain men, buffalo hunters, miners, and cowboys, all interspersed with historical quotations such as this one from President James Polk's 1845 inaugural address: "Our title to the country of the Oregon is clear and unquestionable and already are our people preparing to perfect that title by occupying it with their wives and children."

The museum is open from 8 a.m. to 10 p.m. Memorial Day Weekend through Labor Day and 9 a.m. to 6 p.m. the rest of the year. Museum admission is $1 per person or a maximum of $3 per family. All facilities at the Arch are closed Thanksgiving, Christmas, and New Year's Day.

The Old Courthouse, also on the national monument grounds, dates from 1826 and was the setting for many cases involving slavery, the fur trade, and equal rights, including the 1857 Dred Scott decision.

Visitors may see two free films: "Gateway to the West" and "Time of the West." Tours are available, and all courthouse attractions are free.

The Jefferson National Expansion Monument is located along the Mississippi River on Memorial Drive. Several parking garages are located nearby, including the reasonably priced Arch Garage on the park's north side. Avoid rush hour, particularly during the construction-intensive spring and summer seasons.

The Missouri and Mississippi rivers meet north of St. Louis, and Illinois Highway 3 leads to a view of the confluence. Narcissa Whitman, one of the first white women to travel to the Oregon country, described her 1836 visit to the spot like this: "Twilight had nearly gone when we entered the waters of the great Missouri, but the moon shone in her brightness. It was a beautiful evening. My husband and I went up on the top of the boat to get a more commanding view of the scenery. How majestic, how grand was the scene, the meeting of two such great waters."

Just west of St. Louis on the Missouri River and along Interstate 70, the city of **St. Charles** dates back to 1769, when it was founded by French-Canadians. It later served as Missouri's first capital from 1821 to 1826. But it is possibly most famous for its ties to westward expansion, for it was here that Lewis and Clark camped before starting their trek west.

The Lewis & Clark Center (701 Riverside Drive) is a hands-on museum that traces the explorers' expedition and its discoveries. It is open daily except holidays from 10:30 a.m. to 4:30 p.m. A re-enactment of the Lewis and Clark encampment takes place in St. Charles every third weekend in May. St. Charles' other big annual shindig is Fete des Petites Cotes ("Festival of the Little Hills"), which draws about 300,000 people annually in mid-August.

From St. Charles, continue west on Interstate 70 to Arrow Rock. This small settlement in the middle of Missouri has long been a stopover for people heading west.

SIDETRIP: ST. LOUIS ATTRACTIONS

The Gateway Arch symbolizes St. Louis, and it's also the heart of a vibrant riverfront district offering plenty of urban fun.

Riverboats line the levee, ready to treat visitors to a variety of cruises. The biggest company is Gateway Riverboat Cruises, which operates the Belle of St. Louis, Becky Thatcher, Huck Finn, and Tom Sawyer boats. Even McDonald's has its own riverboat restaurant, complete with a 200-gallon aquarium.

To the north of the Arch, Laclede's Landing marks the spot where Pierre Laclede founded a fur trading post in 1764. Once a decaying industrial district, Laclede's Landing is now one of the most popular spots in St. Louis. Attractions include several antique, rare book, and craft shops, the Wax Museum (720 N. 2nd St.), the National Video Game and Coin-Op Museum (featuring vintage pinball machines, video games and jukeboxes at 801 N. 2nd St.), and an array of restaurants and nightspots, many featuring live music.

Soulard, two miles south of the Arch on Broadway, calls itself "St. Louis' French Quarter" and has one of the city's liveliest music scenes. Check out the great variety of clubs featuring rock, jazz, blues, and even Irish music.

Also near the Arch is Busch Stadium, home of the St. Louis Cardinals. Right next door is the National Bowling Hall of Fame. St. Louis has more than its share of unusual museums: Others include the Dog Museum (1721 S. Mason Road), the Magic House/St. Louis Children's Museum (516 S. Kirkwood Road) and the Dental Health Theatre (727 N. 1st St.). More traditional attractions include the History Museum, St. Louis Art Museum, and St. Louis Science Center, all in Forest Park. The Campbell House (15th and Locust Streets) offers exhibits on early St. Louis and the city's fur trading days.

St. Louis began as a trading post, and shopping continues to play a prominent role in the city's life. Union Station has evolved from a train depot to a popular marketplace with shops, restaurants, and lodging. The St. Louis Centre, also downtown, contains more than 150 stores and restaurants.

The St. Louis Zoological Park, located in Forest Park, is home to more than 3,400 animals, a children's zoo, and one of the nation's largest miniature railroads. The Missouri Botanical Garden spans seventy-nine acres at 4344 Shaw Blvd. and features an English woodland garden, a Japanese garden, and a fragrance garden for the blind. If your botanical tastes run more toward hops and barley, plan a stop at Anheuser-Busch. The brewery at I-55 and Arsenal Street is listed on the National Register of Historic Places and offers free tours Monday through Saturday.

If you happen to be in St. Louis on the second Sunday of the month, consider the architectural tour offered by the local chapter of the American Institute of Architects. The group also offers free self-guiding maps of the city's architectural highlights. Call (314) 621-3484 for information.

Sports-minded visitors should head over to Forest Park. This 1,293-acre preserve in the city's West End offers bicycle rentals, jogging paths, fishing, boating, two public golf courses, and tennis courts. Thoroughbred horse racing is featured mid-March through October at Fairmont Park in nearby Collinsville, Ill.

No description of attractions near St. Louis would be complete without mention of Six Flags Over Mid-America. The mega-amusement park is about thirty miles southwest of downtown, near the Allenton exit off Interstate 44. Water-park fans will enjoy Raging Rivers, located at the opposite end of the St. Louis metro area in Grafton, Illinois.

For more information on St. Louis, call the convention and visitors commission at (800) 247-9791 or write to 10 S. Broadway, Suite 1000, St. Louis, MO 63102.

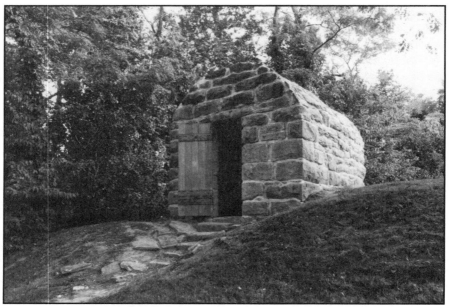

*The "calaboose," or one-man jail, is an attraction at Arrow Rock, Missouri.
Julie Fanselow photo.*

ARROW ROCK, MISSOURI

To the harried city-dweller or suburbanite making this tour, Arrow Rock serves as the first indication that life in some places along the old emigrant trail continues today pretty much as it has for generations. Located thirteen miles northwest of Interstate 70 (take Exit 98 to State Route 41), this town was once home to about 1,000 people. These days, about eighty folks remain.

Settled early in the 1800s, Arrow Rock was originally called New Philadelphia. The town got its current name when two men were vying for the love of a local Indian chief's daughter. The chief said whichever man could shoot an arrow the farthest could marry the young woman. One arrow shot from a sandbar in the Missouri River stuck in the crevice of a bluff above the river, and thus the town was named Arrow Rock.

Beginning in 1821, Arrow Rock became a major jumping-off spot for traders heading down to Santa Fe. In later years, many emigrants passed through the area on their way to the trailheads farther west. The town's population peaked around 1860 but began to dwindle after the Civil War and the decline of traffic on the nearby Missouri River.

Today, Arrow Rock looks much like it did in the mid-1800s. A new state interpretive center explains the town's history, and visitors can see the past up close by walking through town. Historic buildings include the tavern, the old seminary, and a home occupied by by frontier artist George Caleb Bingham from 1837 to 1845. John P. Sites, considered one of the most skilled gunsmiths in the nation, moved here in 1844 and catered extensively to the emigrant trade. His restored shop may still be seen.

A tiny one-room jailhouse—or calaboose—is another point of interest. According to local legend, the only prisoner ever placed in the cell found it so cold that he decided to build a fire. The fire warmed him, but it also woke up several snakes that had been hibernating in the stone building. This understandably unnerved the prisoner, who reportedly raised quite a racket. He was transferred to another jail in nearby Marshall, and the one-room jail was never used again.

About two dozen merchants and innkeepers are doing their best to keep Arrow Rock alive, and the town enjoys thriving tourism, especially in the summer. Shop for everything from antiques and pottery to cast iron cookware and Native American art. The Lyceum Theatre presents professional drama from May through September, and village tours are offered three times daily from Memorial Day through Labor Day and on weekends in the spring and fall.

The Arrow Rock State Historic Site interpretive center is open from 10 a.m. to 4 p.m. Monday through Saturday and from noon to 6 p.m. Sunday. For more information on Arrow Rock, call (816) 837-3231 or 837-3470 or write Friends of Arrow Rock at P.O. Box 147B, Arrow Rock, MO 65320.

SIDETRIP: LAKE OF THE OZARKS

When Missourians play, they frequently head for the Lake of the Ozarks region, located about seventy-five miles southwest of Columbia via U.S. Highways 63 and 54.

Lake of the Ozarks was created in 1931 with the completion of Bagnell Dam. With 58,000 acres of water surface and 1,375 miles of twisting shoreline, the "Big Dragon"—as Lake of the Ozarks is known—has more shoreline than the California coast, all set against the rolling green Ozark hills.

Lake of the Ozarks State Park near Osage Beach is Missouri's largest state park at 17,087 acres. It offers two swimming beaches, boat rentals, horseback riding, fishing, hiking, and 172 campsites. More than 200 resorts are located elsewhere on the lakeshore.

The Ozarks continue on south into Arkansas. Branson, a town near the border, is one of the busiest country music venues in the United States. The Branson area also boasts such family attractions as Silver Dollar City theme park and the Wilderness Safari Wild Animal Kingdom.

For more information on these regions, call the Lake of the Ozarks Visitors Bureau at (800) 325-0213 or the Branson/Lakes Area Chamber of Commerce at (417) 334-4136.

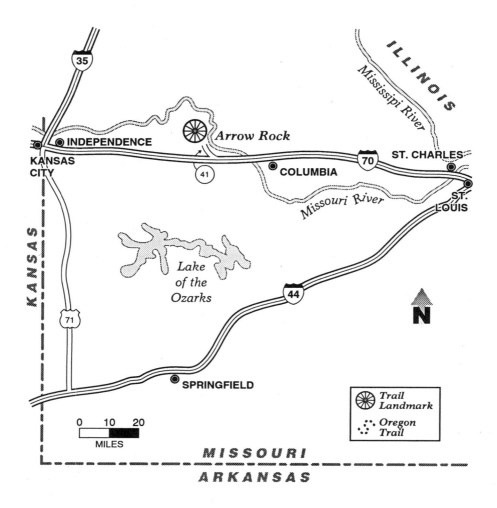

INDEPENDENCE, MISSOURI

The "Queen City of the Trails," Independence today is a somewhat sleepy little city swallowed up by the Kansas City metropolitan area. Aside from the choking traffic on the town's major thoroughfares, it's difficult to believe more than 112,000 people live within the Independence city limits.

But in the mid-19th century, Independence was one brawling, boisterous town. Located just twelve miles from the frontier, the city served as the the major supply depot for travelers heading out on the Oregon, California, and Santa Fe trails. Steamboats from St. Louis docked at Independence Landing to unload people, animals, and wagons. The emigrants would then climb a steep road to the town itself.

During the day, Independence rang with the sounds of people eager to be on the move. Blacksmiths, wagon builders, and other merchants worked feverishly all spring to supply the emigrants. By night, the town continued to bustle as men met in the saloons to talk about Oregon and the coming trip. Campsites dotted the outlying meadows, and in the spring, there would be at least 10,000 oxen grazing in the fields, waiting to move west with the wagon trains.

Independence served as main jumping-off spot for the Oregon Trail until the late 1840s and early 1850s. After that, the Missouri River shifted its course and Westport, St. Joseph, Weston, and Council Bluffs eclipsed Independence as major trailheads. But during the 1840s, at the height of excitement over westward emigration, Independence truly was the "last rest stop in the United States"!

Plenty of Oregon Trail history lives on in Independence, including one of the best trail interpretive sites to be found anywhere: the **National Frontier Trails Center** at 318 W. Pacific Ave., built near "Lot 143," where emigrants topped off their water barrels before heading west.

The center offers a seventeen-minute film that details the origins of all three major trails, the Oregon, California, and Santa Fe. The exhibits allow visitors to both read and hear pioneer diary excerpts and examine artifacts. These halls are filled with human drama, giving names and faces to some of the emigrants and conveying the terrible hardships they endured.

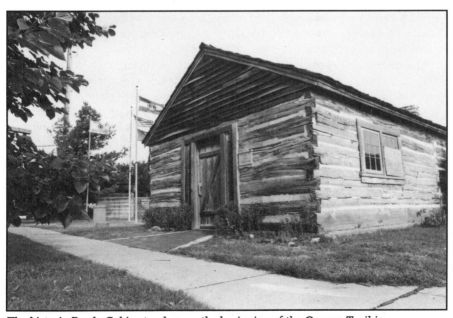

The historic Brady Cabin stands near the beginning of the Oregon Trail in Independence, Missouri. Julie Fanselow photo.

The trails center also is home to an archives and research library containing rare books, letters, and emigrant diaries. Visitors can try to trace their own ancestors' movements across the plains. A statue by Juan Lombardo Rivera commemorates women's roles in westward expansion, and a small gift shop offers tasteful souvenirs ranging from books to replicas of pioneer children's toys.

The National Frontier Trails Center is open weekdays from 9 a.m. to 4:30 p.m. and weekends from 12:30 to 4:30 p.m. except Veterans Day, Thanksgiving, Christmas, and New Year's Day. Admission is $2 for adults 16 to 62, $1.50 for seniors over 63, and fifty cents for children ages 10 to 15. For more information, call (816) 254-0059.

Among other important trail-related sites, **Independence Courthouse Square** was the closest thing to an official starting point the Oregon Trail ever had. It is bordered by Main, Maple, Lexington, and Liberty streets. Nearby, at the corner of Noland and Truman roads, is the **Brady Cabin and Spring,** site of the free-flowing springs that first attracted settlers to Independence.

Every Labor Day Weekend, Independence stages Santa-Cali-Gon Days, a festival marking the city's role as "Queen City of the Trails." The event on Independence Square typically offers Old West foods, carnival rides, staged shootouts, entertainment, and arts and crafts exhibits.

Most folks here say that the remains of Jim Bridger, the famous mountain man and Western guide, are buried in Mount Washington Cemetery, west of Brookside Avenue between Truman Road and U.S. Route 24. Because Bridger was originally buried in Dallas, Missouri, which is now part of Kansas City, some historians believe the remains at Mount Washington aren't actually those of Bridger. Nevertheless, a monument on the site notes his role in opening the West.

Independence is perhaps most famous as the hometown of President Harry S. Truman, and anyone interested in his life and career can choose from a wealth of informative attractions. Truman's courtroom and office are located in the Jackson County Courthouse on the square, where visitors can see a multimedia presentation titled "The Man from Independence." The Truman Library and Museum, at U.S. Route 24 and Delaware Street, includes a replica of Truman's office in the White House.

When not in Washington, D.C., Harry and Bess lived at 219 N. Delaware St. from their marriage in 1919 to his death in 1972, and the home is now designated the Harry S. Truman National Historic Site. Tours are available, but space is limited and tickets must be obtained at the Truman Home Ticket and Information Center at Truman Road and Main Street. Truman held down his first job at Clinton's Soda Fountain & Gifts (100 W. Maple St., on the square).

Other Independence attractions include the unusual spiral-topped temple recently built by the Reorganized Church of Jesus Christ of Latter-day Saints (River Boulevard and Walnut Street); a Mormon Visitors Center run by the regular Church of Jesus Christ of Latter-day Saints

(937 W. Walnut St.); the 1859 Jail & Marshal's Home (217 N. Main St.); the fabulous Victorian-style Vaile Mansion (1500 N. Liberty St.); and the Hair Museum, which displays pictures and jewelry made from human hair—a popular pastime before 1900 (815 W. 23rd St.). Missouri Town 1855, a restored 19th-century community, is located in Fleming Park south of Independence in the city of Blue Springs.

KANSAS CITY AND WESTPORT

Eager to save time and head out across the prairie as soon as possible, some emigrants bypassed Independence in favor of **Westport Landing,** eight miles farther up the Missouri River. The original landing was situated between the present-day Broadway and Heart of America bridges over the Missouri River.

The Westport district, south of downtown via Broadway Avenue, is where Kansas City began and where many emigrants outfitted their wagons before heading west. Today's Westport combines history with a wealth of restaurants, nightclubs, art galleries, and unusual stores. It's a vibrant, interesting area, well worth a few hours of exploring.

Begin a tour of Westport at **Pioneer Park** on the corner of Westport Road and Broadway. Here stands the "Three Trails West" terrazzo mosaic and a statue of three key players in Westport history: freighting magnate Alexander Majors, John Calvin McCoy (who laid out the town in 1834 and was considered the "Father of Kansas City"), and mountain man/frontier scout Jim Bridger.

From the park, head southwest down Westport Road to see two of Kansas City's oldest buildings. The old **Ewing-Boone Store** at 500 Westport Road was operated as an outfitting store from 1851 through 1854. Albert Gallatin Boone (Daniel's grandson) bought out the Ewings and ran a general store on the site until 1859. Like any good businessman, Boone knew the value of "location, location, location"—wagon trains bound for Santa Fe and Oregon passed right by his front door!

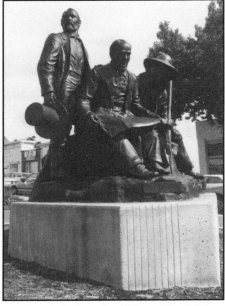

The statue of Alexander Majors, John Calvin McCoy, and Jim Bridger at Westport in Kansas City, Missouri, is a reminder of some of the trail's early pioneers. Julie Fanselow photo.

27

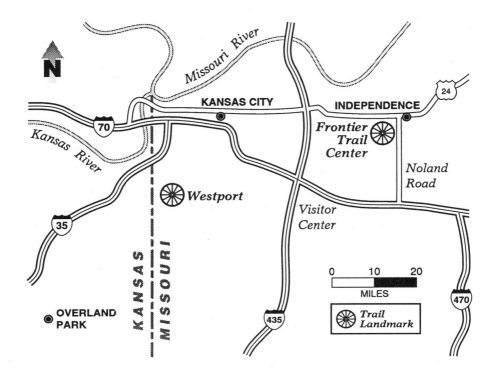

The Ewing-Boone building survived several Civil War-era fires. It was then remodeled by Daniel Meriwether, who ran a grocery and hardware store. A one-story addition was built in 1892. Today, the building houses Kelly's Westport Inn, a friendly, neighborhood-style tavern (and site of KC's premiere St. Patrick's Day Party). Kelly's open door faces the corner of Westport and Pennsylvania, an intersection that is probably the epicenter of Westport and maybe all of Kansas City.

Right next door at 504 Westport Road, Cyprien Choteau and Price Keller built a two-story brick building in 1850. In 1866, Jim Bridger bought the store for $1,000 and had his son-in-law, Albert Wachsmann, run the business. The building is now Stanford & Sons Restaurant, where they serve a Jim Bridger Burger and a cheesecake once voted the best in Kansas City. Farther down the block, visitors can see a movie, play miniature golf, or hear alternative rock 'n' roll at The Shadow.

Westport also played a role in Civil War history. The Battle of Westport was fought here in October 1864, marking the end of Major General Sterling Price's attempt to seize Missouri from Union control. That explains the Confederate and Union "soldiers" still standing watch in second-floor windows at Kelly's Westport Inn.

Because the emigrants followed different routes out of Kansas City, the wagons rolled in many areas. Although there are a few sites in the city where trail scholars insist you can see signs of the wagons' journey (at the Minor Park Golf Course along Red Bridge Road, for example), far better remnants await the traveler farther west.

There are, however, several other historic sites in Kansas City worthy of attention. The **Kansas City Museum** is located at 3218 Gladstone Blvd. in an area of parks, fountains, and mansions, and it has a display and video on westward expansion. The museum is open from 9:30 a.m. to 4:30 p.m. Tuesday through Saturday and noon to 4:30 p.m. Sunday, with admission by donation.

The brick Greek Revival **Wornall House,** at 61st Terrace and Wornall Road, was built by John Wornall in 1858. It served as a hospital for both Union and Confederate casualties during the Civil War. Now fully restored and full of 19th-century textiles, glass, silver, and ironware, Wornall House also offers summer programs for children. It is open from 10 a.m. to 4 p.m. Tuesday through Saturday and 1 to 4 p.m. Sunday. Admission is $2.50 for adults, $2 for senior citizens over 62, and $1 for children under 12.

The **Alexander Majors House** also invites visitors at 8201 State Line Road. Majors began hauling freight from Independence to Santa Fe in 1848. In later years he joined forces with William H. Russell and William B. Waddell to become the top freighting firm on the American frontier. At one point, the company owned 3,400 wagons and 40,000 oxen and employed 4,000 people. The trio also were responsible for starting the short-lived but famous Pony Express overland mail service. The Majors House is open from 1 to 4 p.m. Thursday through Sunday, April through December.

Benjamin Stables at 6401 E. 87th St. offers horseback riding right along the route of the old Santa Fe-Oregon Trail. Fees are $15 for the first hour and $10 for each additional hour.

Emigrants sometimes spent their first night on the trail camping at **Cave Spring,** now a park at the corner of Gregory and Blue Ridge boulevards just west of the suburb of Raytown. New Santa Fe, located near where State Line and Santa Fe roads intersect, was the last "civilized" settlement Oregon-bound emigrants would see before the frontier. From here, about eighteen miles from the starting point in Independence, the pioneers pressed on into what is now Kansas—and what was then the great unknown.

Barely a mile into Indian territory, wagon trains passed the **Shawnee Indian Mission,** near the present-day town of Fairway, Kansas. The mission was established in 1830 by the Rev. Thomas Johnson, and emigrants on their way to Oregon or Santa Fe often stopped to camp in the vicinity. The mission is open from 10 a.m. to 5 p.m. Tuesday through Saturday and 1 to 5 p.m. Sunday. Admission is free.

A very short wagon rut swale—known as the water tower ruts— exists near a water tower at the corner of 79th Street and Delmar in the town of Prairie Village. This was part of the Olathe Cutoff, used by many early emigrants from Westport. Another Olathe Cutoff landmark, **Mahaffie House** at 1100 Kansas City Road, Olathe, served as a wagon and stagecoach stop toward the end of the Oregon Trail's existence.

Emigrants often stayed at **Lone Elm Campground,** at 167th and Elm streets in Olathe. Another possible campsite, simply called Elm Grove, was located about 2.5 miles northwest.

The Oregon and Santa Fe trails split near what is now Gardner. A lone sign on the right fork pointed the way, stating simply, "Road to Oregon." A historical marker about two miles west of town on U.S. Highway 56 notes the parting of the ways, but historians believe the actual split was in Gardner proper, possibly where the elementary school now stands.

This point marks the end of the trail's route through what is now the Kansas City metropolitan area. From here, the Oregon Trail runs north and west near DeSoto and Eudora and on into what is now Lawrence.

SIDETRIP: KANSAS CITY ATTRACTIONS

You wouldn't expect a city in America's heartland to have a decidedly European feel with fountains, broad boulevards, and fine architecture. But Kansas City has long thrived on defying expectations and delighting anyone who pictured it as an overgrown cow town.

Kansas City is, of course, really two geographically and politically separate cities. Kansas City, Missouri (often referred to as KCMO), has a population of about 435,000, while its smaller counterpart in Kansas is home to about 150,000. The seven-county metro area adds nearly a million more people.

Kansas City, Mo., welcomes travelers with a great visitors center right off Interstate 70 at the Harry S. Truman Sports Complex. The friendly people are full of good advice and will even draw a detailed map to help visitors find their way around the area. The Blue Ridge Cutoff heading south of this area was a major route for Santa Fe-bound emigrants

The Truman Sports Complex dominates the view of anyone entering Kansas City from the east. Two huge stadiums with a total of 118,000 seats give a big home-field advantage to baseball's Royals and football's Chiefs. College sports fans won't want to miss the NCAA Visitors Center at 6201 College Blvd. in Overland Park, Kansas, where photos and videos pay tribute to great collegiate athletes.

Recreation enthusiasts can choose from an embarrassment of riches, too. Swope Park's 1,772 acres offer swimming, tennis, golf, fishing, and boating, plus summer concerts by popular entertainers. Worlds of Fun and Oceans of Fun, two popular theme parks, are located thirteen miles north of Kansas City on Interstate 435. Dogs and ponies race at The

Woodlands, a track at 99th Street and Leavenworth Road off of I-435 in Kansas City, Kansas.

Culture plays an equally strong role in Kansas City's life. The Nelson-Atkins Museum of Art (45th and Oak streets) includes fifty-eight galleries and the largest collection of Henry Moore sculptures in the United States. Kansas City was home to artist Thomas Hart Benton, whose home may be toured at 3616 Belleview Avenue.

Visitors who don't get their fill of shopping and entertainment in Westport can check out Country Club Plaza to the south at 47th Street and J.C. Nichols Parkway. Built in 1922, it was the first planned shopping center in the United States. Antique collectors flock to 45th Street and State Line Road, a district with more than fifty antique, arts, and crafts dealers. The open-air City Market at 5th and Walnut streets near the river is a good place to stock up on fresh fruit.

Crown Center just south of downtown is yet another place to eat, party, and shop. Free concerts take place every Friday evening during the summer, and past acts have included such luminaries as the Grateful Dead. (No word as to whether itinerant tie-dye vendors were allowed.) Crown Center also is headquarters for Hallmark Cards, and a free visitors center demonstrates the art and business of greeting cards.

For more information on Kansas City, write the Convention & Visitors Bureau of Greater Kansas City at 1100 Main St., Suite 2550, Kansas City, MO 64105 or call (800)767-7700.

LAWRENCE AND TOPEKA

As the wagon trains rolled on toward present-day Lawrence, the emigrants saw Blue Mound, the first significant landmark on the trail. Although it couldn't compare with the mountains they'd see later, the Blue Mound (today called Mount Bleu) was quite a spectacle to the former flatland farmers, and many climbed it to see the view.

Today, Mount Bleu and the plains are heavily wooded and sure to smash many misconceptions about Kansas. In the Oregon Trail days, however, eastern Kansas conformed more to its barren stereotype. The best view of the Blue Mound is from Kansas Highway 10, which leads into Lawrence as 23rd Street. The rise is about six miles southeast of town.

Many pioneers who passed through the area sent favorable reports back home, and settlement of eastern Kansas started in earnest by the early 1850s. By 1854, Congress had enacted the Kansas-Nebraska Act organizing the Kansas and Nebraska territories and giving them self-determination on the red-hot issue of slavery. The New England Emigrant Aid Company, a group organized to lead Northern resistance against proslavery powers, established the town of Lawrence in September 1854, giving it strong abolitionist sentiment from the start.

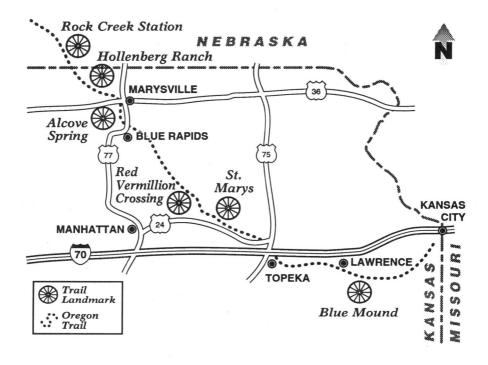

But the pro-slavery faction wasn't ready to concede. In August 1863, Confederate guerrilla William Quantrill led between 300 and 450 western Missourians into Lawrence, where they sacked and burned homes and businesses, left 150 citizens dead and caused some $1.5 million in damage. The renegades no doubt thought they'd had the last word, but Lawrence residents quickly rallied to rebuild their town, and its population more than doubled within the next two years from 2,000 to 5,400. The University of Kansas was founded here in 1866.

Lawrence now has a population of about 65,000 people, and while things are a lot calmer today than during the "Bleeding Kansas" era, the city revels in its youthful population, active cultural scene, and abundant recreational opportunities. Visitors may enjoy strolling the pretty downtown area centered at Massachusetts and Ninth streets, or visiting KU atop Mount Oread. The most popular on-campus attraction, aside from Jayhawk sporting events, is probably Dyche Museum of Natural History, one of the nation's largest. The museum's many interesting exhibits include Comanche, a mounted horse who was the only Seventh Cavalry survivor of Custer's Last Stand.

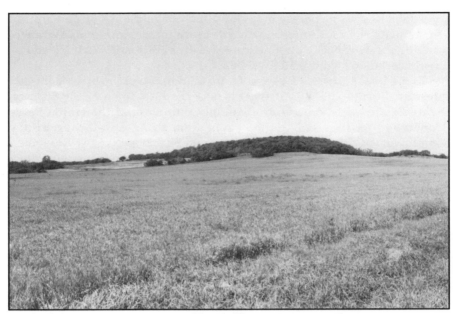

The Blue Mound was a navigational landmark near Lawrence, Kansas.
Julie Fanselow photo.

A National Endowment for the Arts study recently found that Lawrence ranks twelfth in the nation in percentage of artists in the local work force. The result is a strong, varied arts scene that is the envy of cities many times Lawrence's size. Galleries abound, and the community enjoys a full slate of festivals and performances. The Bottleneck at 737 New Hampshire St. is particularly renowned for its eclectic selection of live music. First-run art and independent films show nightly at Liberty Hall, 642 Massachusetts St.

Lawrence takes its recreation seriously, too. Much of it centers around Clinton Lake, four miles southwest of the city via U.S. Highway 40 (which parallels the Oregon Trail). Boating, fishing, swimming, horseback riding, hiking, and camping are all enjoyed on or around the 7,000-acre lake. Clinton Lake and Tuttle Creek near Manhattan are two Kansas state parks that offer "Rent-A-Camp" sites to visitors. For $10 per night, a family of four gets use of a tent (already set up) and campground outfitted with propane stove, lantern, cooler, propane fuel, and cots or sleeping pads. Reservations may be made by mail or by telephone with a major credit card; see the camping section at the end of this chapter for telephone numbers.

Alvamar Golf and Country Club at 1800 Crossgate Drive has a public eighteen-hole course that has been dubbed one of the nation's fifty best.

Lawrence has thirty parks, many of which have plenty of playground gear to keep the kids entertained. For more information on Lawrence, write the Lawrence Convention & Visitors Bureau, 734 Vermont, Lawrence, KS 66044 or call (913) 865-4411.

From Lawrence, the Oregon Trail wandered west near present-day Interstate 70 and U.S. 40. At what is now the little town of Big Springs, the trail split, with some wagons rolling southwest on the Union Ferry Branch and most staying on the main stem straight into present-day downtown Topeka. The branches met again near what is now Rossville.

Although they had already crossed a few small streams with deep banks that made the going difficult, it was in Topeka—after about eight days on the trail—that the emigrants encountered their first real river crossing. Explorer John Fremont, who mapped and described the trail in 1842, described the Kansas River ford as 230 yards wide, with a "swollen, angry yellow turbid current." Sometime that year or soon after, Joseph and Lewis Papin established a ferry to help emigrants across at the price of one dollar per wagon.

By the time they'd reached the Kansas River, the emigrants had gotten to know one another pretty well. It was at this point most wagon trains reorganized, electing a new captain if necessary and cracking down on discipline for the long trip ahead. Jesse Applegate, who made the trip in 1843, described the election process in his journal *A Day with the Cow Column*. At a signal, all would-be captains marched across the prairie. Their fellow emigrants would then run after the candidate of their choice, and the man with the longest "tail" of people would win the job.

Topeka is justly proud of its **Kansas Museum of History,** located at 6425 S.W. Sixth St. near the Kansas River. Here, visitors can see displays telling the natural and human history of the Kansas plains. The museum is open from 9 a.m. to 4:30 p.m. Monday through Saturday and 12:30 to 4:30 p.m. Sunday. Admission is free.

Like Lawrence, Topeka was founded as a free-state stronghold in 1854, and it became the state capital in 1861. Although Topeka saw a few clashes between abolitionists and pro-slavery forces, the city is more famous for a battle fought 100 years later, when the U.S. Supreme Court ruled in favor of school desegregation in Brown v. The Topeka Board of Education. Topeka is also famous for being home to the Menninger Foundation, considered the pre-eminent neuropsychiatric center in the United States.

While in Topeka, tour the state house, which boasts some fine art (including John Steuart Curry's "The Settlement of Kansas" featuring abolitionist John Brown). The Topeka Zoological Park, with its domed tropical rain forest exhibit, is another popular draw. It's located in Gage Park, which sits along Gage Boulevard between 6th and 10th streets. The Combat Air Museum, located at Forbes Field south of the city, has

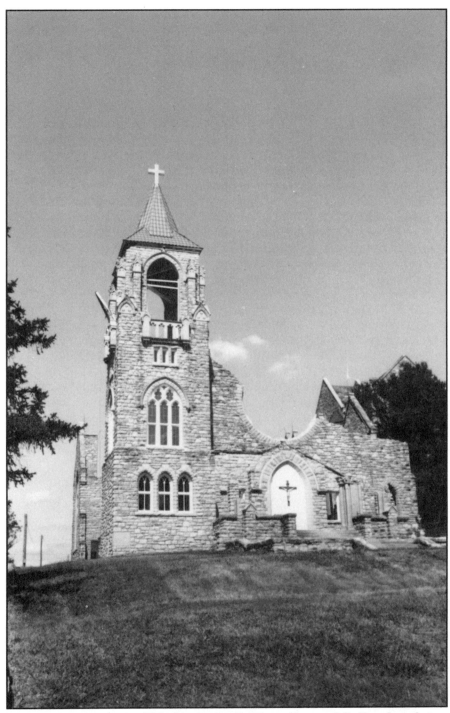

St. Marys Mission was established in 1848 at St. Marys, Kansas. Julie Fanselow photo.

examples of aeronautical technology from all 20th-century U.S. military conflicts. For more information, call the Topeka Convention and Visitors Bureau at (800) 235-1030.

ST. MARYS

From Topeka, take U.S. Highway 75 north two miles to U.S. Highway 24, and head west. Again, the highway parallels the old trail right through the small towns of Silver Lake (which bills itself "The Fastest Growing City in the Country"), Rossville and St. Marys. Watch your speed on this stretch, particularly in Silver Lake.

St. Marys is an interesting little gem of a town rarely mentioned in guidebooks. Many Oregon Trail emigrants camped here since fresh horse and oxen were available. But the town's main claim to fame was the **St. Marys Mission,** established in 1848 among the Pottawatomie Indians. The Jesuit missionaries had lived with the tribe in eastern Kansas for a decade and followed the Indians here when the federal government forced the tribe's relocation. The Indian Pay Station Museum, at First and Mission streets, has exhibits on Pottawatomie history.

On the north side of Highway 24, you'll find St. Marys College, which still operates as a preparatory school for boys. A boulder on campus marks the site of the mission's log cabin cathedral, the first erected between the Missouri River and the Rocky Mountains. A chapel of more recent vintage remains on campus, but it was seriously damaged by fire in 1978. You can still see the outline of a once-beautiful stained glass window. The school hopes to rebuild the Immaculata chapel and double its seating capacity to about 700 without altering the original design. Restoration efforts began in 1990.

RED VERMILLION RIVER CROSSING

West of St. Marys, drive through Belvue, population about 200. Once past Belvue, watch for Onago Road (No. 509) on the right-hand side. Turn right and drive north for three miles, then turn left on Oregon Trail Road. Follow it about a mile to the **Louis Vieux Gravesite,** in a cemetery high on a hill.

Vieux, of mixed French and Pottawatomie ancestry, ultimately became chief of the tribe. He moved to the area in 1847 or 1848 and established a toll bridge over the river. Many Oregon Trail emigrants used the bridge, which cost $1, and Vieux made as much as $300 a day during the peak travel season. He added to that income by selling hay and grain to the pioneers.

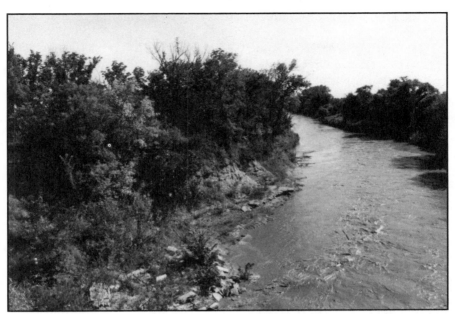

Some emigrants forded the turbulent Red Vermillion River, but many travelers paid to cross a toll bridge instead. Julie Fanselow photo.

Nearby, visitors can see the beautiful Red Vermillion. Birds swoop down its canyon as wind rushes through the trees on the river bank. Well off the beaten path, the crossing gives the modern traveler a chance to breathe deeply and forget the urban rush, for it will be a long time before next encountering anything that could be called a traffic jam.

Emigrants liked this area, too, for it offered plenty of water, wood, and grass, which all would be in short supply in the months ahead. They could also marvel at the Louis Vieux elm, the largest American elm tree in the world at 99 feet high. About 130 years old at the time of the Oregon Trail, it may still be seen near the west side of Vermillion bridge.

All was not well here in May 1849, however. That spring, an outbreak of Asiatic cholera choked the emigrant camps, killing dozens of travelers. More than fifty people in one train died and were buried near the river. A small, fenced-in cemetery preserves three headstones, and one still bears the inscription "T.S. Prather, May 27, 1849."

Follow the backroad four miles southwest to Kansas Highway 99 at Louisville. At this point, travelers can stay closest to the original trail by taking Highway 99 north for thirty-three miles to Frankfort. Pick up Kansas Highway 9 at Frankfort and drive fourteen miles west to Blue Rapids. Or, from Louisville, drive three miles south on Highway 99 to Wamego on U.S. Highway 24, and take Highway 24 to Manhattan, a good overnight stop.

Manhattan, a town of some 37,000 folks, is home to Kansas State University. Tuttle Creek State Park, a popular and productive fishing spot with hundreds of campsites, is just north of town. **Fort Riley** is also nearby. Established in 1852, the outpost was situated midway between the Oregon and Santa Fe trails and was designed to provide protection to travelers on both routes.

Travelers taking the route through Manhattan will find the intersection of U.S. Highways 24 and 77 about fifteen miles northwest of the city. Highway 77 runs north to Blue Rapids and Alcove Spring, the next major site along the Oregon Trail.

SIDETRIP: OTHER TRAILHEADS

Independence and Westport were the best-known jumping-off spots for the Oregon Trail. But other settlements along the Missouri River—notably St. Joseph and Weston, Missouri, and Council Bluffs, Iowa—rose to prominence as trailheads, too.

Joel Palmer recommended St. Joe highly in his emigrant guidebook, writing "For those emigrating from Ohio, Indiana, Illinois, and Northern Missouri, Iowa, and Michigan, I think St. Joseph the best point; as by taking that route the crossing of several streams (which at the early season we travel are sometimes very high) is avoided." By 1849, about twenty steamboats visited St. Joseph each day, and most of the boats were filled with people bound for the West.

An exhibit titled "Wagons West" at the **St. Joseph Museum** tells of the city's role in the westward migration. It explains how travelers often waited two or three days to have their wagons ferried across the Missouri River so they could roll west. The museum, located at 11th and Charles streets, is in the 1879 Wyeth-Toole Mansion. St. Joe is also home of the Pony Express, and a museum celebrating the "lightning mail" service may be found at 914 Penn St, where the horses were housed.

Weston, Missouri, no longer sits on the river, but in 1853 it was the state's second largest river port and a major embarkation point for Oregon Trail travelers. Today, this town twenty miles south of St. Joe is best known for its many pre-Civil War homes and for the nation's oldest and smallest distillery, the McCormick Distilling Company, founded in 1856 by stagecoach magnate Benjamin Holladay. The facility is located southeast of Weston on County Road JJ, and tours are available.

What is now known as Council Bluffs, Iowa, was a major Mormon community called Kanesville in the 1840s. Members of the Church of Jesus Christ of Latter-day Saints built the town in 1846, only to abandon it a few years later at the behest of church president Brigham Young,

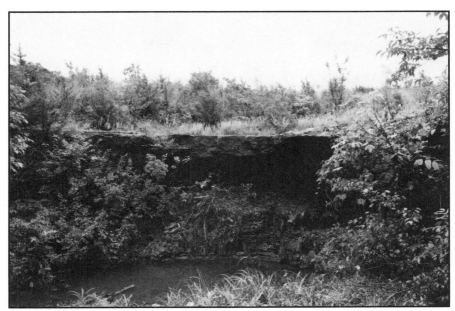

The obscure Alcove Spring was a pleasant rest spot before crossing the Big Blue River. Julie Fanselow photo.

who summoned them to the new Mormon settlement near Utah's Great Salt Lake. When the Mormons left, Kanesville's population dropped abruptly from 8,000 to 1,000. But the city soon became a key rail center, and it continued its importance to overland emigrants as a natural gateway to the Platte River Valley, pathway across the plains.

Leavenworth, Kansas, was not on the main Oregon Trail but the town still played a role in westward expansion. **Fort Leavenworth** was established in 1827 to protect traffic on the Santa Fe Trail. In later years, other emigrants passed through the area, and in 1856 the freighting firm of Majors, Russell, and Waddell made Leavenworth its headquarters. The Frontier Army Museum at Fort Leavenworth explains the military's role in opening the West.

ALCOVE SPRING

Long one of the most celebrated stops on the Oregon Trail, **Alcove Spring** has fallen into obscurity. For years, the spot was an official Kansas state park, but vandalism forced its closure to the public. It may now be visited only by permission, which should be obtained in advance by writing or calling the owner, Stella Hammett of Blue Rapids. Her address is 413 E. 5th St., Blue Rapids, KS 66411.

To reach the site, turn west just before the Blue River bridge south of Marysville. Follow this road south for about five miles, and keep an eye out for a row of knee-high posts on both sides of the road (not far from the railroad tracks). This is the entrance to Alcove Spring. Park by the gate and look eastward beyond several large boulders. At the 2 o'clock position rests a small monument. The path to the spring is to the right of this marker.

Emigrants typically arrived at Alcove Spring in late spring and often had to camp several days to wait for the Big Blue River's early season runoff to subside so they could ford safely at Independence Crossing, just a quarter-mile away. But it was a fine place to be delayed a while. Many emigrant diaries noted the cold, clear rushing water, the tall green grass, and the beautiful wildflowers blooming in profusion near the spring. The only problem were the mosquitoes, which some emigrants insisted were big as turkeys. But mountain man Joe Meek tried to put that rumor to rest by reporting that "the biggest one I saw was no larger than a crow." Alas, the pesky critters still throng around the spring today, and insect repellent is a must.

Among those who camped here were the Donner Party of 1846, which would later be trapped by an early blizzard in the high Sierras of California. Edwin Bryant, a Donner Party member, is said to have named Alcove Spring, and he and fellow traveler Byron McKinstry carved that legend on the rock surrounding the spring.

James Frazier Reed also was traveling with the Donner Party. Reed, who survived the Donner trek, carved his initials in a boulder at the spring. His mother-in-law, "Grandma" Sarah Keyes, was 70 years old, blind and deaf. She was traveling west in hopes of rejoining her son, who had emigrated to Oregon two years earlier. But she died at Alcove Spring, a merciful thing considering the horrors the Donner Party would face farther west. The Daughters of the American Revolution marker commemorating her journey reads: "God in his love and charity has called in this beautiful valley a pioneer mother."

Grandma Keyes was buried here, but not before relatives clipped and saved a lock of her hair. Amazingly, the lock survived the whole trip, even the Donner Party's trek across the Sierras. When eight-year-old Patty Reed was rescued from a snow cave in California, she was found clutching her grandma's lock of hair in her small hand.

Kansas storms are legendary, and it was near here that Francis Parkman encountered one of the worst he would see along the trail in 1846. "Scarcely had night set in when the tumult broke forth anew," he wrote. "The thunder here is not like the tame thunder of the Atlantic coast. Bursting with a terrific crash directly over our heads, it roared over the boundless waste of prairie, seeming to roll around the whole circle of the firmament with a peculiar and awful reverberation. The lightning flashed all night, playing with its livid glare upon the neighboring trees, revealing the vast expanse of the plain, and then leaving us shut in as if by a palpable wall of darkness."

From Alcove Spring, return to Highway 77 and drive north to Marysville, a cordial little town offering free RV parking in its city park. Facilities include electric hook-ups, a dump station, and restrooms (but no showers). Marysville also has a small selection of motels and restaurants.

Marysville got its name from the wife of frontier merchant Frank Marshall, who ran an emigrant ferry across the Big Blue River. This was where travel along the original Independence road and the later St. Joseph road converged. A woman whose name was lost to history offered this description of the scene near Marysville: "It was a grand spectacle when we came for the first time, in view of the vast migration, slowly winding its way westward over the broad plain. The country was so level we could see the long trains of white-topped wagons for many miles...it appeared to me that none of the population had been left behind. It seemed to me that I had never seen so many human beings before in all my life."

Marysville was also a major town along the Pony Express route. An original Pony Express home station and museum may be visited at 106 S. 8th St, and a sculpture on Highway 36 leading out of Marysville tells more about the mail service. Follow Highway 36 west to Kansas Highway 148. Turn north and drive 4.5 miles to Kansas Highway 243. Turn right. The Hollenberg Ranch is one mile east.

SIDETRIP: THE PONY EXPRESS

The histories of the Oregon Trail and the Pony Express are closely intertwined. Each took place during the same era in American history, following roughly the same route across the plains of Kansas and Nebraska. Each involved elements of excitement, romance, and danger. And many road ranches built to serve the emigrant trade later became Pony Express stations.

The Pony Express was founded in April 1860 by Russell, Majors, and Waddell, the same trio who ran the Overland Stage. Their new corporation, the Central Overland and Pike's Peak Express, promised mail delivery between St. Joseph, Mo., to Sacramento, Calif., in a mere ten days, about half the time of the fastest stagecoaches.

The entrepreneurs advertised for courageous young men to ride the mail across the 1,800-mile route and back again. The Pony Express recruiting poster specified the company's preferences: "Young skinny wiry fellows not over eighteen. Must be expert riders willing to risk death daily. Orphans preferred." Eighty such young men rode the Pony

Express at a time, forty going west, forty going east. Their pay was $50 each month, plus meals.

A series of way stations, where riders changed horses, was established about every ten miles along the route. "Home" stations, where riders could sleep, were set up about every fifty miles.

The first ride from St. Joe to Sacramento took nine days and twenty-three hours. The fastest run—carrying President Lincoln's inaugural address to an eager Western audience—took just seven days and seventeen hours. At first, the Pony Express run was made just once weekly, but that quickly grew to twice weekly and then daily.

In his book *Roughing It*, Mark Twain described the delight of seeing a Pony Express rider from his stagecoach: "We had a consuming desire, from the beginning, to see a pony-rider, but somehow or other all that passed us and all that met us managed to streak by us in the night, and so we heard only a whiz and a hail, and the swift phantom of the desert was gone before we would see him in broad daylight."

Finally, however, the stage party spotted a rider in time. "Every neck is stretched further, and every eye is strained wider. Away across the endless dead level of the prairie a black speck appears across the sky, and it is plain that it moves. Well, I should think so! In a second or two it becomes a horse and rider, rising nearer—growing more and more defined—nearer and nearer, and the flutter of the hoofs comes faintly to the ear. Another instant a whoop and hurrah from our own upper deck, a wave of the rider's hand, but no reply, and man and horse burst past our excited faces, and go winging away like a belated fragment of a storm."

Although popular, the Pony Express was expensive. Initially, it cost five dollars to send a letter weighing a half-ounce, but the price was later reduced to a dollar. Operational expenses, however, did not diminish. In all, the service required 500 horses, 200 men to care for the animals en route, and vast amounts of grain to feed the animals. Russell, Majors, and Waddell lost $100,000 during the "lightning mail" system's eighteen months of operation.

The Express' history was fraught with physical as well as economic peril. Indians frequently burned and looted Pony Express stations, which were highly visible reminders of the white man's increasing presence in the West. Riders also had to contend with blizzards, stream crossings, and hot desert sand. Despite these dangers and discomforts, only one mail delivery was ever lost.

The Pony Express ended in October 1861 when completion of a transcontinental telegraph system made it possible to deliver messages in seconds, not days. A service that only months before had seemed new, exciting, and incredibly fast had been rendered obsolete. But the Pony Express lives on in the American imagination and at a few well-preserved landmark stations strung out across the nation.

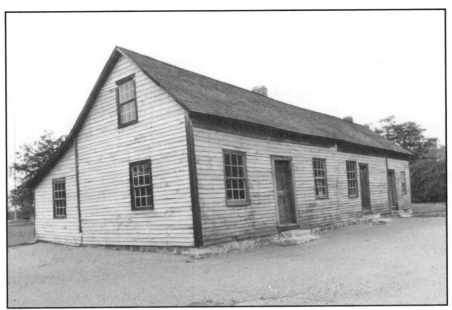

The Hollenberg Ranch, sometimes called the Cottonwood Station, provided meals, lodging, and livestock for emigrants. Julie Fanselow photo.

HOLLENBERG RANCH

The **Hollenberg Ranch** is another often-overlooked site along the Oregon Trail, although that may change soon: In 1992, Senator Robert Dole of Kansas recommended that the ranch be turned into a major federal interpretive site for the entire Pony Express route.

Gerat H. Hollenberg had traveled the Oregon Trail as a gold miner in 1849. He later moved to Kansas and ran a general store in Marshall County before moving west to Washington County, where he established a business a few hundred yards northwest of Cottonwood Creek. The Hollenberg Ranch Station, as it was named, included a general store, post office, and tavern, as well as the Hollenberg home.

Hollenberg knew what he was doing when it came to locating his business. Countless emigrants passed through the valley, camping at Cottonwood Creek and relying on Hollenberg Ranch—sometimes called Cottonwood Station—for meals, lodging, food, clothing, and livestock. In 1860, Hollenberg Ranch became a station for the Pony Express, and it is today the only remaining unaltered Pony Express Station standing on its original site in the entire United States. In 1991, repairs were made to stabilize the building without altering its historical character, and every-thing was put back to within an eighth-inch of where it had been. In the meantime, an archaeological dig unearthed many souvenirs of the ranch's heyday. Some of the artifacts are on display.

Duane Durst has farmed in Washington County for many years and now serves as a guide at Hollenberg Ranch. He hopes to see a day when the ranch can be interpreted just as it was in the 1850s and 1860s. Until then, visitors can stroll through the ranch house, look at exhibits, and picnic out on the lawn overlooking the Cottonwood Creek valley. With a little imagination, today's travelers can almost see the hundreds of white-topped wagons that crowded the area 150 years ago.

Hollenberg Ranch is open from 10 a.m. to 5 p.m. Tuesday through Saturday and from 1 to 5 p.m. Sundays. Admission is by donation. On the last Sunday each August, Hollenberg Ranch holds a Pony Express Festival featuring Oregon Trail and Pony Express re-enactments, buffalo burger barbecues, living history demonstrations, and a circuit-rider church service.

Hollenberg Ranch is just a few miles from the Nebraska border. Return to Kansas Highway 148 and head north into the Cornhusker State.

LODGING

GREATER ST. LOUIS, MISSOURI

Best Inns of America, (618) 397-3300, I-64 and Route 157 (Caseyville, Illinois), $41.

Best Western Camelot Inn, (800) 528-1234, I-220 and Illinois Highway 111N (Pontoon Beach, Illinois), $37.

Days Inn at the Arch, (314) 621-7900, 333 Washington Ave., $59-$99.

Hampton Inn, (800) HAMPTON, I-270 Exit 26B (Florissant), $49-$54.

Holiday Inn-West Airport, (800) HOLIDAY, I-270 and St. Charles Rock Road (Bridgeton), $55.

Knights Inn, (314) 291-8545, 12433 St. Charles Rock Road (Bridgeton), $38-$41.

Motel 6, (314) 427-1313, 4576 Woodson Road, $39.

Super 8 Motel, (800) 843-1991, 12705 St. Charles Rock Road, (Bridgeton), $41.

ST. CHARLES, MISSOURI

Country Inn by Carlson, (800) 456-4000, 2750 Plaza Way, $45.

Econo Lodge, (800) 446-6900, I-70 Exit 227, $39.

Red Roof Inn, (800) 843-7663, I-70 Exit 227, $37.

COLUMBIA, MISSOURI

Budget Host Crossways Inn, (800) 456-1065, I-70 Exit 127, $24-$36.

Guesthouse Inn, (314) 474-1408, I-70 Exit 128A, $44.

Drury Inn, (800) 325-8300, 1000 Knipp St., $56-$62.

Eastwood Motel, (800) 274-3278, 2518 Business Loop 70E, $33-$44.

University Inn, (314) 449-2401, Broadway and Short streets, $34-$45.

BOONVILLE, MISSOURI

Comfort Inn, (800) 4CHOICE, I-70 and Route 5, $43-$53.

The Homestead Motel, (816) 882-6568, Highway 5.

ARROW ROCK, MISSOURI

Airy Hill Inn, (816) 837-3458.

Borgman's Bed & Breakfast, (816) 837-3350, $40-$45.

Cedar Grove Bed & Breakfast, (816) 837-3441, $50-$60.

DownOver Bed & Breakfast Inn, (816) 837-3268, $40-$60.

Miss Nelle's Bed & Breakfast, (816) 837-3280, $45.

INDEPENDENCE, MISSOURI

Arthur's Horse & Carriage House Bed & Breakfast, (816) 461-6814, 601 W. Maple.

Howard Johnson-East, (800) IGO-HOJO, 4200 S. Noland Road, $47-$62.

Red Roof Inn, (800) 843-7663, 13712 E. 42nd Terrace, $37-$43.

Queen City Motel, (816) 254-1077, 11402 E. U.S. 24, $25-$35.

Serendipity Bed & Breakfast, (816) 833-4719, 403 N. Delaware, $45.

Super 8, (800) 843-1991, I-70 and Noland Road, $32-$44.

Woodstock Inn Bed & Breakfast, (816) 833-2233, 1212 W. Lexington Ave., $45-$50.

GREATER KANSAS CITY, MISSOURI/KANSAS

American Motel, (816) 763-0600, 11801 Blue Ridge Blvd. Extension, $36-$40.

Best Western Overland Park Inn, (800) 528-1234, 7200 W. 107th (Overland Park, Kansas), $60.

Days Inn, (800) 325-2525, 9630 Rose Hill Road (Lenexa, Kansas), $38-$42.

The Embassy on the Park, (816) 471-1333, 1215 Wyandotte St., $50-$64.

Fairfield Inn, (800) 228-2800, 4401 W. 107th (Overland Park, Kansas), $49.

Howard Johnson Convention Center, (800) IGO-HOJO, 610 Washington St., $49-$79.

Motel 6, (816) 228-9133, I-70 Exit 20 (Blue Springs), $34.

Ramada Inn South, (800) 228-2828, 6701 Longview Road, $45.

LAWRENCE, KANSAS

Best Western Hallmark Inn, (800) 528-1234, 730 Iowa Street, $40-$42.

Eldridge Hotel, (913) 749-4512, 701 Massachusetts St., $74-$82.

Jayhawk Motel, (913) 843-4131, 1004 N. 3rd.

Halcyon House Bed & Breakfast, (913) 841-0314, 1000 Ohio.

Holiday Inn, (800) HOLIDAY, I-70 West Lawrence Exit, $62-$86.

Quality Inn University, (800) 221-2222, 6th and Iowa.

Westminster Inn, (913) 841-8410, 2525 W. 6th St., $38.

TOPEKA, KANSAS

Comfort Inn, (913) 273-5365, 1518 S.W. Wanamaker Road, $42.

Days Inn, (800) 325-2525, 1510 S.W. Wanamaker Road, $42.

Heritage House Bed & Breakfast, (913) 233-3800, 3535 S.W. 6th, $60-$125.

Holiday Inn-West, (800) HOLIDAY, 605 Fairlawn Road, $54-$60.

Sunflower Motel, (913) 234-5591, 624 N. Highway 24.

TOPEKA, KANSAS (CONT.)

Super 8 Motel, (800) 843-1991, 10th Avenue and Wanamaker Road, $40.

Topeka Plaza Inn, (913) 266-8880, Highway 75S and I-470.

MANHATTAN, KANSAS

Best Western Continental Inn, (800) 528-1234, 100 Bluemont, $40-$52.

Days Inn, (800) 325-2525, 1501 Tuttle Creek Blvd., $38-$52.

Motel 6, (913) 537-1022, 510 Tuttle Creek Blvd., $29-$35.

Ramada Inn, (800) 228-2828, 17th and Anderson, $57-$61.

Super 8 Motel, (800) 843-1991, 200 Tuttle Creek Blvd., $41.

MARYSVILLE, KANSAS

Best Western Surf Motel, (800) 528-1234, 2005 Center St., $34-$47.

Thunderbird Motel, (913) 562-2373, Highway 36 West, $28-$36.

CAMPING

GREATER ST. LOUIS

Babler Memorial State Park, (314) 458-3813.

North Greater St. Louis KOA, (618) 931-5160, 3157 West Chain of Rocks Road, Granite City, Ill.

St. Louis West KOA, (314) 257-3018, Interstate 44 bus loop, Allenton, Missouri. Kamping Kabins available.

WENTZVILLE, MISSOURI

Pinewoods Park, (314) 327-8248, Interstate 70 Exit 208.

JONESBURG, MISSOURI

Jonesburg KOA, (314) 488-5630, Interstate 70 Exit 183.

DANVILLE, MISSOURI

Graham Cave State Park, (314) 564-3476, Exit 170 to County Road TT.

Kan-Do Kampground, (314) 564-7993, Exit 170 to Service Road TT.

BOONVILLE, MISSOURI

Bobber Campground, (816) 882-6334, I-70 and Highway B.

ARROW ROCK, MISSOURI

Arrow Rock State Historic Site, (816) 837-3330, State Route 41.

CONCORDIA, MISSOURI

Spacecraft Campground, (800) 762-2389, West Outer Road.

INDEPENDENCE, MISSOURI

Lake Jacomo Campground, (816) 229-8980, Colbern Road, Blue Springs.

Longview Reservoir, (816) 229-8980, View High Drive, Lees Summit.

LAWRENCE, KANSAS

Clinton State Park, (913) 842-8562, U.S. Highway 40 West. Rent-A-Camp sites available; call for information.

Lawrence KOA, (913) 842-3877, northeast of town on U.S. Highway 40. Kamping Kabins.

TOPEKA, KANSAS

Perry State Park, (913) 289-3449, 16 miles northeast on State Route 237.

KOA of Topeka, (913) 246-3419, U.S. Highway 24, Grantville.

Lake Shawnee Campground, 3435 SE Eastedge Road.

MANHATTAN, KANSAS

Tuttle Creek State Park (913) 539-7941, Highway 24 North. Rent-A-Camp sites available; call for information.

MARYSVILLE, KANSAS

City Park, (913) 562-3101, 10th and Walnut.

RESTAURANTS

GREATER ST. LOUIS, MISSOURI

Arciela's, (314) 776-5900, 2501 S. 9th at Victor. Mexican food.

Bogie's, (314) 241-9380, 809 N. 2nd. Specialties include prime rib.

Casa Gallardo, several locations in St. Louis area, including 12380 St. Charles Rock Road, (314) 739-5700. Mexican food, Sunday brunch.

Charlie Gitto's Pasta House, (314) 436-2828, 207 N. 6th. Popular restaurant for the budget-conscious.

Kennedy's 2nd Street Company, (314) 421-3655, 612 N. 2nd St. Casual dining with live music. Children welcome.

Lettuce Leaf Restaurant, (314) 241-7773, 107 N. 6th St., Salad, soups, pizza, sandwiches.

Norton's Cafe, (314) 436-0828, 808 Geyer. Cajun and Creole specialties.

Old Spaghetti Factory, (314) 621-0276, 727 N. 1st St. Italian food in converted 1874 factory building.

ST. CHARLES, MISSOURI

Madison's Cafe, (314) 928-7355, 73 Charleston Square. Italian and American dishes.

Old Country Buffet, (314) 947-0122, 2867 I-70 Service Road.

COLUMBIA, MISSOURI

Carlos Garcia's, (314) 442-1184, 909 Business Loop 70E. Northern Mexican food.

Heritage House Smorgasbord, (314) 443-4567, 1010 I-70 Drive S.W.

Katy Station, (314) 449-0835, 402 E. Broadway. Dine in converted boxcars and train station.

Old Plantation House, (314) 443-6212, 4515 Highway 763N. Rural setting with steak and seafood.

The Original Bobby Buford Restaurant, (314) 445-8647, I-70 and Stadium Boulevard. Steak and seafood.

BOONVILLE, MISSOURI

Bobber Restaurant, (816) 882-6334, I-70 and Highway B. Open 24 hours.

ARROW ROCK, MISSOURI

Arrow Rock Ice Cream Emporium, (816) 837-3337. Sandwiches, desserts.

The Evergreen Restaurant, (816) 837-3251, Highway 41. Fine dining in restored 1840s home. Call for reservations.

The Old Schoolhouse Cafe, (816) 837-3331. Breakfast and lunch.

The Old Tavern, (816) 837-3200, Main Street. Country-style cooking.

INDEPENDENCE, MISSOURI

Applebee's Neighborhood Grill and Bar, (816) 795-7799, 2035 Independence Center. Family style food.

The Black-Eyed Pea, (816) 478-3545, 14001 E. U.S. 40. Homestyle cooking.

Courthouse Exchange, (816) 252-0344, 113 W. Lexington. Midwest cuisine.

The Rheinland Restaurant, (816) 461-5383, 208 N. Main St. German cuisine.

Winstead's, (816) 252-9363, 1428 S. Noland Road. Steakburgers, fountain specialties.

GREATER KANSAS CITY, MISSOURI/KANSAS

Casa de Tacos, (913) 342-6226, 19th and Central (Kansas City, Kansas). Authentic Mexican food.

Corner Restaurant, (816) 931-6630, 4059 Broadway. Westport's favorite breakfast spot.

D'Bronx, (816) 531-0550, 3904 Bell St. New York-style deli fare.

Frontier Steak House, (913) 788-9159, 9338 State Avenue (Kansas City, Kansas).

Furrs Cafeteria, (816) 765-3110, I-435 and Bannister Road.

Gates Barbecue, (816) 923-0900, 4707 Paseo and five other locations. Often voted K.C.'s best.

Papagallo, (913) 831-0928, 4208 Rainbow Blvd. Italian, Mediteranean and vegetarian cuisine.

Paradise Diner, (913) 894-2222, Oak Park Shopping Center (Overland Park, Kansas). "Cross-cultural cusine."

Remington's, (816) 737-4760, in the Adam's Mark Hotel, I-70 at Sports Complex. Steaks, seafood, wild game.

Westport Flea Market, (813) 931-1986, 817 Westport Road. Famous burgers.

LAWRENCE, KANSAS

American Bistro, (913) 841-8349, 7th and Massachusetts. Regional cuisine, fresh seafood, Sunday brunch.

Don's Steak House, (913) 843-1110, 2176 E. 23rd St.

Free State Brewery, (913) 843-4555, 636 Massachusetts. Micro-brewery and restaurant, all ages welcome.

Paradise Cafe, (913) 842-5199, 728 Massachusetts. Creative menu, fresh fish, bakery.

Plum Tree, (913) 841-6222, 2620 Iowa St. Oriental food.

Teller's, (913) 843-4111, 746 Massachusetts. Pizza, Italian food featuring organic ingredients.

TOPEKA, KANSAS

Annie's Place, (913) 273-0848, 4014 Gage Center Drive. Casual dining featuring fresh-baked breads and desserts.

Casa, (913) 266-4503, 3320 S. Topeka Blvd. Mexican and American food.

Carlos O'Kelly's, (913) 266-3457, 3425 S. Kansas Ave. Mexican-American cafe.

Old Country Buffet, (913) 273-8393, 1801 S.W. Wanamaker Road (in the Westridge Mall). Wide selection of food.

Por'e Richard's, (913) 233-4276, 705-707 Kansas Ave. Casual dining downtown.

WAMEGO, KANSAS

The Friendly Cooker, (913) 456-8460, 520 Lincoln.

MANHATTAN, KANSAS

Country Kitchen, (913) 776-6301, 420 Tuttle Creek Blvd. Reliable family fare.

Kearby's, (913) 539-1332, 8385 Highway 24. Family dining with frequent buffets.

Sirloin Stockade, (913) 776-0516, 325 E. Poyntz

Valentino's, (913) 537-4350, 3003 Anderson. Pizza and more.

MARYSVILLE, KANSAS

Fiesta La Grande, (913) 562-5395, 308 Center.

Koester House Restaurant, (913) 562-2279, 908 Elm.

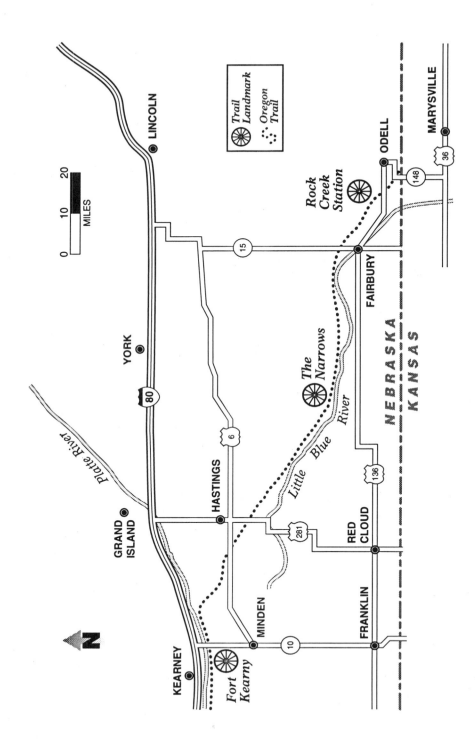

MILES
0 10 20

Trail
Landmark
Oregon
Trail

LINCOLN

YORK

80

6

15

HASTINGS

GRAND
ISLAND

Platte River

KEARNEY

Fort
Kearny

MINDEN

10

281

FRANKLIN

RED
CLOUD

136

Little Blue River

The
Narrows

Rock
Creek
Station

FAIRBURY

ODELL

148

36

MARYSVILLE

NEBRASKA
KANSAS

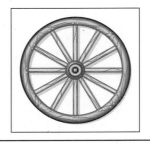

CHAPTER FOUR

THE PLATTE RIVER ROAD: NEBRASKA

"As we wended our way up the valley of the Platte, one could look back for miles and miles on a line of wagons...with vari-colored wagon covers, resembling a great serpent crawling and wriggling up the valley."

—William Thompson, overlander

ROCK CREEK STATION

It is true the Platte River accompanied the emigrants most of their way across what is now Nebraska. But to reach the Platte, the travelers stayed close to the Little Blue River, moving northwest across what is still a sparsely settled area of American plains.

The first stop in Nebraska on today's trail is **Rock Creek Station State Park,** and although it is somewhat off the beaten path, it is well worth a visit. The Nebraska parks department has done a great job of interpreting this site, and there's something to capture everyone's interest.

After entering Nebraska, Highway 148 jogs east then north to the small town of Odell. Pick up Nebraska Route 8 here and drive west to Endicott. Rock Creek Park is 2.75 miles north then one mile east.

Rock Creek was a popular camping spot for trappers, traders, and emigrants even before a station was officially established. Although Rock

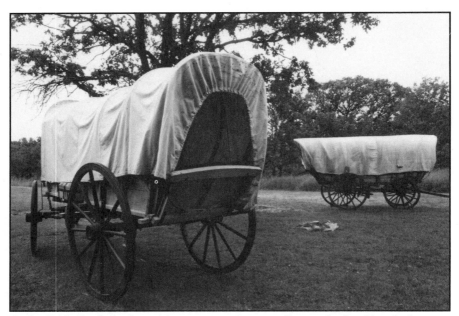

At the Rock Creek Station, visitors can see wagon replicas and other historical reconstructions. Julie Fanselow photo.

Creek's steep-sloped crossing was difficult, the area offered good spring water, fuel, and grass for grazing. Among the most notable early visitors to the area were John Fremont and his scout, Kit Carson, who camped in the area in 1842.

The first recorded settlers came to the area in 1856, and S.C. and Newton Glenn built Rock Creek Station on the west side of the creek in 1857, operating the stage station and trading post for several years until David McCanles took over. Deciding the West Ranch lacked sufficient water, McCanles built a new ranch on the creek's east side and enlarged it a few years later. McCanles also built the toll bridge that saved travelers from having to make the difficult creek crossing. He charged from ten cents to fifty cents per wagon, depending on ability to pay and the size of the wagon load.

Although Rock Creek Station was a major stopping point on the Oregon Trail, the Overland Stage route, and the Pony Express, it is perhaps best known as the place where James Butler "Wild Bill" Hickok launched his gunfighting career by killing McCanles and two hired men on July 12, 1861, in a gruesome incident witnessed by McCanles' twelve-year-old son, Monroe. Hickok had been on the ranch since the spring of that year, working as a hand for the Overland Stage; McCanles had nicknamed him "Duck Bill" because of Hickok's nose and prominent upper lip. The shootings took place when McCanles attempted to collect a long-overdue payment on the East Rock Creek Station from Horace Wellman, who managed the site for the Overland Stage Co. Early in July 1861, Wellman said he would travel to Nebraska City to attempt to get the money from the stage company. He arrived back at the ranch July 12. A Nebraska state pamphlet on the incident relates the day's events like this:

"When Mrs. Wellman came to the door, McCanles asked if her husband was there. When she replied that he was, McCanles demanded that he come out. She informed him that he would not, adding to McCanles' anger and suspicion. He then told Mrs. Wellman that if her husband would not come out, he would come in and drag him out. With that, Hickok stepped to the door."

"Hickok's sudden appearance disconcerted McCanles and heightened his anger. He figured that either the company was bankrupt and could not pay the money due or Wellman had collected it and planned to cheat him out of it. He had mentioned these suspicions to his family many times during the preceding month.

"Being a former sheriff and with no law close at hand, McCanles determined on quick action. Powerfully built and unafraid of any man, he would repossess the station by simply throwing the occupants off the premises by physical force.

"Having no quarrel with Hickok, McCanles asked him if they hadn't always been friends. Hickok assured him this was so. Evidently sensing that something was amiss and in a play for time, McCanles asked Hickok for a drink of water. While drinking he apparently saw something, and handing the dipper back to Hickok, hurried to the other door. While he was crossing the room, Hickok ducked behind the calico curtain that divided the room.

"Although his quarrel was with Wellman, McCanles now had Hickok to contend with as well. At the same time, Hickok must have realized that both he and Wellman were no match for the powerful McCanles. As he reached the other door, McCanles called for Hickok to come out and fight it out fair if he had anything against him.

"In reply to McCanles' challenge, Hickok, from his hiding place behind the curtain, took aim with the very rifle McCanles had left behind to defend the station. Deliberately and in cold blood, he shot McCanles through the heart. It was a tactic that he would use successfully throughout his gunfighting career."

Hearing the commotion, McCanles' cousin, James Woods, and his friend, James Gordon, ran toward the cabin. They, too, were shot dead by Hickok, who later tried to claim the killings were in self-defense. His account gained credibility through publication in dime-novels and magazines. Hickok was acquitted of the killings when young Monroe McCanles was not allowed to testify at Hickok's trial in Beatrice. He went on to become one of the West's most notorious characters, finally meeting his demise at age 39 in a Deadwood, S.D., saloon.

Before exploring Rock Creek Park, take a good look at the land here. Much of it has never been tilled. The grasses grow high, and many species of birds and flowers thrive. This is an excellent example of basically unaltered prairie, and it is as beautiful in its own way as the Rocky Mountains or the desert Southwest.

Rock Creek Station State Park took shape only in recent years. During the 1960s, the Nebraska Game and Parks Commission set about purchasing the land that encompassed the two old road ranches. At that time, no traces could been seen of the East Ranch, the West Ranch, or the toll bridge that connected the two. By the early 1980s, archaeological teams arrived to unearth clues on the whereabouts of the ranch buildings and how life had been lived there. Since then, several ranch buildings and the toll bridge have been reconstructed.

At the visitor center, exhibits tell of the Oregon Trail, the Pony Express, and the Hickok connection. Don't miss the aerial photo showing nearby trail ruts.

A short path from the visitor center to the west and east ranches parallels some of those ruts. The path is lined with dozens of native grasses in individually planted plots, all identified and labeled. At the West Ranch, you can view several wagon replicas. The blue one served as the official Nebraska centennial statehood wagon in 1967.

Crossing the toll bridge to the East Ranch, listen for the clanking of metal from a blacksmith's shop. With a little luck, visitors might catch Roy Kappel at work on the anvil. A former bookkeeper from Elk Creek, Nebraska, Kappel became interested in blacksmith work when he started rebuilding wagons. He's been working at Rock Creek for more than a decade now, and all the products of the blacksmith shop are used in the park's reconstruction efforts.

Rock Creek Station's visitor center is open from 9 a.m. to 5 p.m. daily during the summer and from 1 to 5 p.m. weekends during May, September, and October. Admission is by a $2 daily permit. Annual permits that cost $10 also are available. For more information, call (402) 729-5777.

Weather permitting, Rock Creek offers short wagon rides from 10 a.m. to 4 p.m. Wednesday through Sunday all summer long. The cost is just $1.50 per person. A campground and horse camping facilities are available too.

Fairbury, about six miles west of Rock Creek, is a pleasant town of 4,300 people. Its beautiful city park includes a playground, pool, and lots of shade.

From Rock Creek the trail cuts northwest to the Platte River, meeting it near Fort Kearny, our next stop. There are several ways to get to Fort Kearny from Fairbury. Each route is fairly complicated, so we'll take them one at a time:

Option One (About 150 miles): Drive U.S. Highway 136 west to Red Cloud, then U.S. Highway 281 north to Hastings. From Hastings, take U.S. Highway 6 to Minden and Nebraska Highway 10 to Fort Kearny. Deshler, a small town along Highway 136 seven miles west of Hebron, offers free camping in its city park.

This region is most famous as the girlhood home of Pulitzer Prize-winning writer Willa Cather, who later wrote about the Nebraska prairie in many of her novels. Red Cloud attractions include the Willa Cather Memorial Prairie, a 610-acre tract of native grassland five miles south of town on Highway 281; the Willa Cather Historical Center on Webster Street; and the Willa Cather home at Third Avenue and Cedar Street.

Option Two (About 160 miles): Take Nebraska Route 15 north to U.S. Highway 6, which jogs northeast a few miles before meeting Interstate 80. From here, it's 110 miles to Kearney.

A thirty-mile round-trip detour east on Nebraska Highway 4 (some ten miles north of Fairbury) leads to the Homestead National Monument. This 160-acre claim was filed by Daniel Freeman, who settled on it during the Civil War under the provisions of the Homestead Act of 1862. He was one of more than a million homesteaders who settled the Great Plains about the same time that travel on the Oregon Trail was slowing to a trickle. The site includes a century-old log cabin, a restored country school, and a pioneer farm equipment display, as well as a 1.5-mile trail through the tall grass prairie.

Other attractions along this route include short detours to the Hastings Museum or the Stuhr Museum of the Prairie Pioneer in Grand Island. Situated on an island in a manmade lake, the latter is considered one of the best museums in the region. Its exhibits include a re-created nineteenth-century railroad town and the birthplace of actor Henry Fonda. Two popular state recreation areas—Mormon Island and Windmill—also lie along this route. Each offers camping, picnicking, swimming, and non-motorized boating.

Option 3 (About 140 miles): Take U.S. Highway 136 west to Hebron, then U.S. Highway 81 north to Fairmont. Follow U.S. Highway 6 west through Minden to Hastings, and then Nebraska Highway 10 north to Fort Kearny.

Hastings is home to the Fisher Rainbow Fountain in Highland Park, and to the Hastings Museum, which features natural history, a "People on the Plains" exhibit, and the J.M. McDonald Planetarium. And Minden is home to Harold Warp's Pioneer Village (see sidebar).

No main roads parallel the Oregon Trail through this region of Nebraska. The pioneers followed the Little Blue River, which today still winds its way northwest from Fairbury past the small towns of Powell, Hebron, Oak, Angus, and Deweese. West of Oak, the emigrants traveled through a stretch known as The Narrows, where the space between the river bank and surrounding bluffs left only enough room for a single wagon.

An average of fifteen people died each mile along the Oregon Trail, and most of their graves were quickly lost to history. But southeast Nebraska has several that may still be seen. George Winslow succumbed to cholera in 1849 and was buried northwest of Fairbury. A monument marking the site is embedded with Winslow's original headstone. It is on private property, but visitor may ask permission to enter; check at the Rock Creek Station visitor center for directions.

Susan Hail was buried a few miles northwest of present-day Kenesaw, on a windswept hill near where the pioneers entered sandhill country and got their first glimpse of the Platte River. One version of Hail's 1852 death maintained that she drank from a spring poisoned by Indians, but Gregory Franzwa wrote in *The Oregon Trail Revisited* that it's more likely she ingested polluted water from a well sunk too close to a campground or a buffalo wallow.

SIDETRIP: PIONEER VILLAGE

For miles away in every direction, travelers see the signs: "Visit Pioneer Village," "Nebraska's No. 1 Attraction," "See How America Grew."

Minden, Nebraska, is indeed synonymous with Harold Warp's Pioneer Village. Warp, who made big money as the inventor of Flex-O-Glass and other plastics, got the idea for Pioneer Village when the old country school he had attended as a child in Minden went up for sale in 1948. Warp has said he didn't plan to build the village, that it just evolved. But as has been said elsewhere in the Midwest, "If you build it, they will come," and five million people have.

Practically a city unto itself, Pioneer Village (with twenty-eight buildings and its own RV park, motel, and airstrip) boasts 50,000 historical items that depict America's progress since 1830. The collection includes 350 antique autos, 100 antique tractors, twenty historic "flying machines," original art by the likes of John James Audubon and William H. Jackson, toys, trolleys, bicycles, buttons, golf clubs, bath tubs, and the list goes on and on.

Poring over the massive collections at Pioneer Village can easily eat up several days, but visitors can enjoy a stop at the site even if with only an hour or two to spare. Pioneer Village is open daily from 8 a.m. to dusk. Admission, $5 for adults and $2.50 for kids ages 6 to 15, is good for any number of consecutive days. For more information, call (800) 445-4447 or (308) 832-1181 in Nebraska.

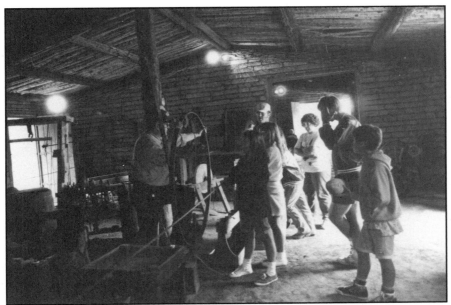

The blacksmith's shop at Fort Kearny offers a glimpse of what life was like in the mid-1800s. Julie Fanselow photo.

FORT KEARNY

Fort Kearny was built in 1848 to protect travelers on the Oregon Trail. It was the first of six major forts the pioneers would pass on their way west, and the only one built specifically for their safety. Fort Kearny also served as a Pony Express and Overland Stage station, an outfitting post for many Indian campaigns, and the seat of military and civil government in the area. The fort was named for Col. Stephen Watts Kearny, who was the first to suggest that a chain of military posts be built from the Missouri River to the Rocky Mountains to protect the Oregon migration.

Congress agreed. In addition to authorizing the forts, it created an Oregon battalion of mounted volunteers to help patrol the route. The first Fort Kearny was established at Table Creek (present-day Nebraska City, near the banks of the Missouri River in the state's southeast corner), but the location was later shifted 197 miles west.

Fort Kearny was a busy place, particularly during the peak years of California gold rush migration. One traveler who visited Fort Kearny described its impact like this: "The emigrant...sees once more the evidence of civilization and refinement, the neat and comfortable tenements of the officers, the offices and stores, all remind him of home, and as he

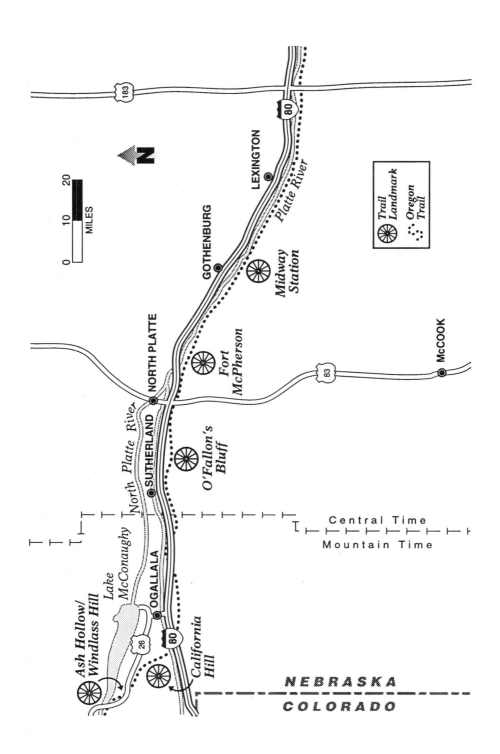

N

0   10   20
MILES

Trail
Landmark

Oregon
Trail

183

80

LEXINGTON

GOTHENBURG

Platte River

Midway
Station

NORTH PLATTE

Fort
McPherson

McCOOK

83

SUTHERLAND

North Platte River

O'Fallon's
Bluff

Lake
McConaughy

Central Time

Mountain Time

Ash Hollow/
Windlass Hill

OGALLALA

26

80

California
Hill

NEBRASKA

COLORADO

looks aloft at the masthead, where the stars and stripes are proudly waving to the breeze, he fully realizes he is still protected, still inhabits America."

War Department records show that 30,000 people passed through the fort during one eighteen-month period in the late 1840s. A decade later, the march was still on: One report indicated that 800 wagons rolled through on a single day just before the Civil War. Business slacked off after the war, and Fort Kearny was abandoned as a military post in 1871.

After the fort closed, its buildings were torn down to make way for homesteaders. Soon, the earthworks of the fortifications and the big cottonwood trees, still visible around the old parade grounds, were all that remained. In 1928, the Fort Kearny Memorial Association was formed. It purchased the forty acres where most of the old buildings stood. But it wasn't until 1960 that the Nebraska Game and Parks Commission set about interpreting the site.

Today, **Fort Kearny State Historical Park** boasts beautiful tree-shaded grounds. A stockade replica has been erected, but visitors will learn that the original wasn't even in place until 1864, a time when Oregon Trail traffic was tapering off but Indian "depredations" were on the rise.

Elsewhere on the grounds, the outlines of many fort buildings are still visible. A self-guided walk offers a glimpse of what life was like at the facility. Especially interesting are the posted excerpts from an 1864 inspection. Officials were praised, for example, for planting cedar, cottonwood, and elm trees near the hospital for the pleasure of convalescing patients.

Modern-day Fort Kearny also includes a recreated blacksmith's shop and an interpretive center with fort artifacts and a slide show. The center is open from 9 a.m. to 5 p.m. daily all summer and 1 to 5 p.m. weekends in May, September, and October, but the grounds stay open from 8 a.m. to 8 p.m. year-round. Admission is by $2 daily permit. A "Fort Kearny Stampede," celebrating the area's role in the nineteenth-century emigration, is held at the historical park each July. For more information on park activities, call (308) 234-9513.

Two settlements near Fort Kearny—Doby Town two miles west and Dog Town eight miles east—catered to soldiers at the post and sold them goods and services that were banned or otherwise unavailable at the fort. Civilians too sometimes visited these frontier tourist traps. Of Doby Town, one writer of the era said: "The townspeople are mostly frontiersmen who settled there for the sole purpose of preying on those who traveled the Oregon Trail. The population consisted chiefly of men; about two dozen permanent inhabitants, mostly gamblers and saloon keepers, some loafers...and a few women of well-known reputation."

Fort Kearny State Recreation Area is next door to Fort Kearny Historical Site. This pleasant park features a 1.8-mile hike-bike trail that parallels the Oregon Trail, along with camping, fishing, swimming, boating (non-power or electric motors), and picnicking. It's a popular spot, so expect crowds and arrive early in the evening to obtain a campsite.

Just a few miles from Fort Kearny, the city of Kearney is one of the most interesting towns in Nebraska. Home to about 25,000 people and a 10,000-student University of Nebraska branch campus, the town has more than its share of culture, recreation, and other diversions, not to mention a wide range of motels and restaurants. The Kearney Visitors Bureau will send information to those who write to P.O. Box 607, Kearney, NE 68848 or call (800) 227-8340 (or (800) 652-9435 in Nebraska).

Fort Kearney Museum, 311 S. Central Ave., exhibits artifacts from all over the world and offers glass-bottom boat rides on a clear spring-fed lake. Railroad buffs will enjoy the Trails and Rails Museum at 710 W. 11th St., and motorheads will thrill to Chevyland U.S.A., located west of town at I-80's Exit 257. Cabela's, the outdoor outfitting catalog company, has a showroom store on Highway 30 east of Kearney featuring one of the state's largest aquariums, trophy game, and fish displays, and a "bargain corner" full of discontinued catalog merchandise. Cooks will probably want to pay a visit to Morris Press on east Highway 30, which has published fund-raising cookbooks for groups in all fifty states. They offer one free cookbook per visitor; additional copies are $2 each.

Kearney's main claim to recreational fame is probably the Prairie Hills Golf and Ski Club, eleven miles north of I-80 Exit 272 on Nebraska Route 10. This site actually does double duty as a ski hill in winter and an eighteen-hole golf course after the spring thaw.

Nine of Nebraska's I-80 rest areas feature sculptures that were put in place during the state's celebration of the U.S. Bicentennial in 1976. One of the most interesting installations is located just west of Kearney. George Baker's 7,200-pound stainless steel "Nebraska Wind Sculpture" floats lazily on a lake, reflecting the blue sky and golds and greens of the surrounding plains.

Speaking of landscape, Kearney is in Nebraska's famous sandhills region, which runs north of the Platte River roughly from Grand Island west to Lewellen. The sandhills are still covered with rich native grass and act as natural reservoirs for irrigation water. The rises at the south edge of the Platte River valley are clay hills, not sandhills, and they are primarily used for grazing.

This also was the area in which the pioneers first caught up with the Platte, which would guide them for hundreds of miles into present-day Wyoming. A natural thoroughfare for travelers, the Platte offered good supplies of grass and water. Emigrants marveled at the shallow, muddy waterway, calling it "a mile wide and an inch deep" or "too thick to drink and too thin to plow." One traveler said it appeared to be flowing bottom-side up. However it is described, the Platte certainly is one of the most distinctive-looking rivers in North America.

Oregon Trail pioneers weren't the only travelers who passed through the Platte River valley. Even today, about a half-million birds—eighty percent of the world's sandhill crane population—rest and feed in central Nebraska during their annual migration north to Canada and Alaska. Popular places to watch the cranes include Fort Kearny and Mormon Island state recreation areas. The birds are usually seen only during a six week span in March and April.

MIDWAY STATION

Travelers along I-80 will see signs encouraging them to stop and see the Pony Express station in Gothenburg, and it is worth a visit. But **Midway Station**, just a few miles south of the Gothenburg interchange (Exit 211) is much less known and at least as interesting.

The station in Gothenburg's Ehman Park was built in 1854 four miles east of Fort McPherson along the Oregon Trail and moved to its present location in 1931. Midway Station, on the other hand, is sitting on the exact same plot of land where it was built about 1850. It is believed to be the only Nebraska Pony Express station still standing on its original site.

Midway Station can be found by driving two miles south of the Gothenburg exit. Turn left at the "96 Ranches" sign, and follow the ranch road back to the station.

This land has been in the family of Janice Williams Gill since the 1870s. (It was owned by Pat Mullaly during the time of the Oregon Trail and the Pony Express.) Gill's husband, Larry, says the ranch grew up around the old station, which was named "Midway" since it sat halfway between Plum Creek and Fort McPherson. After the station was built, a two-story house was added to quarter the ranch foreman and his family. The house burned down in 1959, but the station was unharmed except for smoke damage.

Nevertheless, some restoration has been done. A cement floor was installed to help preserve the building, and shingles have replaced the old sod roof. Other than that, Midway Station stands pretty much as it was during the nineteenth century. Visitors are welcome, but ask the Gills for permission. "We really like to have visitors," Larry Gill says. "It's a little justification for all the money we spend to maintain this place."

Back in Gothenburg, the Ehman Park station is open daily from 8 a.m. to 9 p.m. during the summer, and from 9 a.m. to 6 p.m. during May and September. Horse-drawn carriage rides are offered about every twenty minutes. For more fun, stop by Lake Helen on the north edge of town. Rent a paddleboat or canoe, do some fishing, picnic, and see what is possibly Nebraska's only covered bridge. Camping is available in adjacent Lafayette Park.

Fort McPherson National Cemetery is between Gothenburg and North Platte, four miles south of the Maxwell interchange (Exit 190). The cemetery sits near the site of Cottonwood Springs, which was a major Oregon Trail campsite, trading post, and Pony Express station. A fort was established nearby in 1863 to protect the final waves of traffic along the Oregon Trail during a period of increased Indian hostilities. Emigrant wagon trains sometimes banded together here so that they could face the rest of the way west with increased strength and safety in numbers.

Southeast of the cemetery, a monument on the right side of the road marks the site of the fort's flagstaff. The monument also pays tribute to the Seventh Iowa Cavalry, Civil War veterans who were the first troops stationed at Fort Cottonwood, which was renamed Fort McPherson in 1866. The fort was disbanded in 1880, but its headquarters building may still be seen at the Lincoln County Historical Museum in North Platte.

Valley View Guest Ranch near Maxwell offers swimming, guided trail rides, hayrides, fishing, campsites, and housekeeping cabins. The ranch sits two miles south of the Maxwell exit, then a half-mile west and another half-mile south. Call (308) 582-4320 for more information.

Travelers interested in Native American life may want to take a side trip to the Dancing Leaf Earth Lodge at Stockville, Nebraska, about fifty miles south of Gothenburg via Nebraska highways 47, 23, and 18. Hosts Les and Jan Hosick offer a variety of programs ranging from two-hour tours to overnight stays, all by appointment. For more information, write the lodge at P.O. Box 121, Stockville, NE 69042, or call (308) 367-4233.

SIDETRIP: NORTH PLATTE AND THE BUFFALO BILL RANCH

The Oregon Trail stayed south of present-day Interstate 80 through what is now Lincoln County, but North Platte—the county seat and one of the region's largest cities—still proves fascinating to anyone interested in the lore of the American West.

North Platte's main attraction is probably Buffalo Bill State Historical Park. Located 3.5 miles northwest of town via Highway 30, the park preserves the home of William F. "Buffalo Bill" Cody, one of the West's most colorful characters.

Cody was born in 1846 in Iowa and moved to Kansas with his family in 1853. By age eleven he was driving oxen for fifty cents a day; by age fourteen he became a Pony Express rider, one of the youngest in the ranks. He once rode 322 miles in twenty-one hours and forty minutes, exhausting twenty horses along the way.

Cody was too young to enlist when the Civil War began, but he did serve the Union as a ranger, dispatch bearer, and scout. In 1864, he enlisted in the Kansas Volunteer Infantry and served until the end of the war.

Buffalo were a constant sight along the Oregon Trail during the 1840s and 1850s. Emigrant diaries tell of wagon trains being surrounded by stampeding herds, and buffalo meat was a staple in the pioneers' diet as they crossed the Plains. Indians, too, relied heavily on the great beasts for everything from food to clothing. But by the end of the nineteenth century, the great herds were gone. Blame it on guys like "Buffalo Bill," who is said to have killed 4,280 buffalo in eight months while employed to hunt meat for workers on the Kansas Pacific Railroad.

Cody settled in the North Platte area in 1878 and built the home at his Scout's Rest ranch in 1886. This was the heyday of his Wild West Show, which traveled across North America and even into Europe. All of Cody's many exploits are described in detail at the park, and visitors can even see the Wild West Show via rare film footage shot by Thomas Edison in 1898. Other activities include horseback riding and buffalo stew cookouts Wednesday through Friday evenings July through mid-August.

Buffalo Bill State Historical Park may be visited from 8 a.m. to 5 p.m. year-round. The Cody home is open from 10 a.m. to 8 p.m. Memorial Day through Labor Day, as well as from 9 a.m. to 5 p.m. weekdays and 1 to 5 p.m. weekends in May, September and October. Admission is by $2 daily vehicle permit or $10 annual state parks permit. Call (308) 535-8035 for more information.

The four-day Buffalo Bill Rodeo kicks off each year's celebration of Nebraskaland Days, one of the state's largest festivals. Typically held the third week in June, Nebraskaland Days also features parades, top-name country entertainment, barbecues, dances, and old-style shoot-outs. For those who miss Nebraskaland Days but still crave some bronc-bustin' action, catch the Rough Riders Rodeo nightly through July and August.

Bailey Yard, focal point of the Union Pacific system, is a must for railroad fans. Three miles west of North Platte on Front Street, the yard is the largest rail classification center in the United States. A railroad museum at the city's Cody Park is home to Union Pacific's Challenger 3977, the world's largest steam locomotive and the only one in its class on display anywhere. Other Cody Park attractions include swimming, tennis, picnic grounds, and summer carnival rides for the kids. For more information on North Platte, stop by the Convention & Visitors Bureau at 502 S. Dewey or call (800) 955-4528.

It's about 130 miles north of North Platte via U.S. Highway 83, but canoeists will not want to miss the Niobrara River. Ranked as one of the nation's best paddling streams, the Niobrara features pine-dotted canyons and waterfalls accessed via the Fort Niobrara National Wildlife Refuge area east of Valentine. Call the Valentine Visitor Center at (800) 658-4024 for more information.

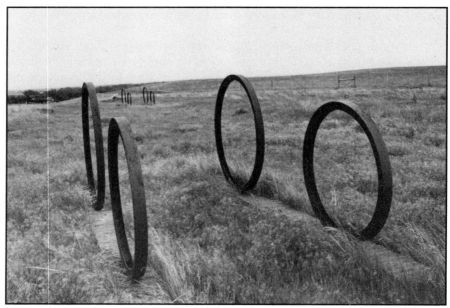

Iron hoops resembling wagon wheels mark the trail at O'Fallon's Bluff.
Julie Fanselow photo.

O'FALLON'S BLUFF

The truth is, a modern traveler could get a fairly good idea of what the Oregon Trail was all about without ever leaving the interstate highway. Many rest areas along the route have excellent displays interpreting the great emigration. One of the best of these is along I-80 in Nebraska at **O'Fallon's Bluff,** about twenty minutes past North Platte.

There's only one minor problem: The bluff is located on the eastbound side of the interstate. If you're traveling west, as most folks tracing the Oregon Trail will do, you will need to backtrack slightly to get there. Leave I-80 at Exit 159, the Sutherland interchange. Get back on the highway eastbound; the rest area is just two miles away.

Although it isn't officially part of Nebraska's I-80 "sculpture garden without walls," the O'Fallon's Bluff deserves honorary membership. Walk to the east edge of the rest area to see several historic markers describing the Oregon Trail. Nearby are several sets of large iron hoops resembling wagon wheels, all poised to roll off across the prairie. Very faint ruts are visible along the ground below.

O'Fallon's Bluff was a landmark to mountain men and pioneer alike. The bluff came so close to the Platte River that emigrant wagons were forced to travel single-file over the route.

From here, the emigrants continued along the south side of the Platte to the Lower California Crossing near present-day Brule, Nebraska. Modern westbound travelers should backtrack three miles eastbound to the Hershey interchange (Exit 164), then continue west on I-80 to Ogallala.

There are a few other sites of interest along or near the Platte in south-central Nebraska. Sutherland State Recreation Area, south of Exit 159 on Nebraska Highway 25, is popular with anglers, boaters, and swimmers. For a break from the interstate, take Highway 30, which parallels I-80 through some of the finest sandhill country and through small towns including Hershey, Sutherland, Paxton, and Roscoe.

If the family's fixin' for a meal at this point, consider stopping in Paxton at Ole's Big Game Lounge and Grill. Established by Rosser O. "Ole" Herstedt one minute after Prohibition ended on Aug. 9, 1933, Ole's now is most famous for its collection of trophy game, all taken by Ole himself during five decades of hunting on every continent. More than 200 mounts are on display, including a 1,500-pound, eleven-foot polar bear taken by Ole in 1969 in the Chukchi Sea off Sibera. He once turned down an offer of $50,000 for the bear.

Ole's menu features steaks, buffalo burgers, seafood, and chicken. What with its decor, Ole's—even more so than most places in cattle country—is probably not the best rest stop for ardent vegetarians and animal-rights activists. But for everyone else, it's a Nebraska institution, open from 8 a.m. to 1 a.m. Monday through Saturday and 10 a.m. to 10 p.m. Sunday.

One additional note: Don't forget to set watches back one hour at the Lincoln-Keith County line, where the Mountain Time zone begins. This is the first of two time zones that give westbound Oregon Trail travelers an extra hour for exploration and fun! It's also another sure sign of officially having passed from the Midwest into the West.

SIDETRIP: OGALLALA AND LAKE MCCONAUGHY

Sitting at the gateway to Nebraska's "panhandle," Ogallala is the jumping-off spot for western Nebraska's Oregon Trail landmarks: Courthouse Rock, Chimney Rock, and Scotts Bluff. Aside from that, Ogallala and its neighbor to the north, Lake McConaughy, combine to offer a region full of activities and recreation.

Named for the Oglala Tribe of the Dakota Sioux, Ogallala nonetheless is more famous for cowboys than for Indians. From 1875 to 1885, Ogallala reigned as "Queen of the Cowtowns," the end of the Texas Trail. From here, cattle driven north from Texas were shipped via the Union Pacific to ranges all over the northern Plains.

Ogallala had another nickname, too: "Gomorrah of the Plains." Much of the town's rowdy reputation came courtesy of cowboys, who flooded Ogallala's saloons and gambling parlors to celebrate the end of their cattle drive. Attracted by all the commerce and commotion, Ogallala soon became a haven for unsavory characters, many of whom are now buried in Boot Hill at 10th and West C streets.

A historical marker at the cemetery confirms that many buried there "came by running afoul of the law—some for stealing another man's horse. Others were killed by re-fighting the Civil War or for questioning the gambler's winning hand. In July of 1879, three cowhands were buried in a single day, victims of the sheriff's guns. Another man, 'Rattlesnake Ed,' was buried here after he was shot down over a nine dollar bet in a Monte game in the Cowboy's Rest, a local saloon."

Today's Ogallala—a community of about 5,000 people—is considerably more tame than the town of yore. But touches of the frontier live on. Front Street is the hub of activity, offering such attractions as the family-style Crystal Palace Revue, a free Cowboy Museum, and nightly "shoot-outs" all summer long. Ogallala also has a good selection of restaurants and recreational attractions including golf, miniature golf, bowling, roller skating, and swimming.

Lake McConaughy sprawls nine miles north of Ogallala via Nebraska Highway 61, and it must be seen to be believed. With 105 miles of sandy beach, the 35,000-acre "Big Mac"—Nebraska's largest reservoir—caters to boaters, water and jet skiers, sailboarders, anglers, swimmers, campers, and sunbathers. As with all Nebraska state parks, a $2 vehicle entry permit is required and may be purchased from the state game commission or from lake-area concessionaires (who charge twent-five cents extra). Stop by any local business for an orientation map.

Lake McConaughy is famous for its fish, and its waters have yielded state-record salmon, trout, striped bass, walleye, and tiger muskie. All anglers age 16 and over need a license; three-day non-resident permits cost $8.

Several full-service campgrounds dot the area around Lake McConaughy and its small neighbor to the east, Lake Ogallala. But visitors can also camp free in many areas around both lakes. Among the choicest locations: Spring Park/Otter Creek, located at Gate 12; Martin Bay, at Gate 1; and the west side of Lake Ogallala. Cabins are available in several locations too, as are services including boat rentals, diving equipment, showers (there are no shower facilities in the state park camping areas), and guide services for anglers and hunters.

"Big Mac" was created in 1941 with the completion of the Kingsley Dam, which impounded the North Platte for irrigation and power generation. When completed, it was the world's second-largest hydraulic dam, and it produces nearly 100 million kilowatt hours of electricity each year, the equivalent of 175,000 barrels of oil.

Central Nebraska Public Power & Irrigation offers free tours of the dam from 11 a.m. to 5 p.m. (Mountain Daylight Time) weekdays and from 9 a.m. to 5 p.m. holidays and weekends. Tours meet at the south end of the dam.

For more information on Ogallala or Lake McConaughy, contact the Ogallala/Keith County Chamber of Commerce at 206 East A St, Ogallala, NE 69153, or call (800) 658-4390.

CALIFORNIA HILL

Ready for an adventure? This fact isn't mentioned on many maps or tourist information leaflets, but western Keith County, Nebraska, is home to some of the finest Oregon Trail ruts to be seen anywhere along the route. At **California Hill**, visitors can walk where the wagons rolled and see the emigrant caravans' impact on the land—traces that haven't vanished even a century and a half later.

To get to California Hill, drive west on U.S. Highway 30 from Ogallala to Brule. Before continuing, take a look at the South Platte River, which may be seen from the road bridge leading to the I-80 interchange south of town. It was in this general location that the emigrants

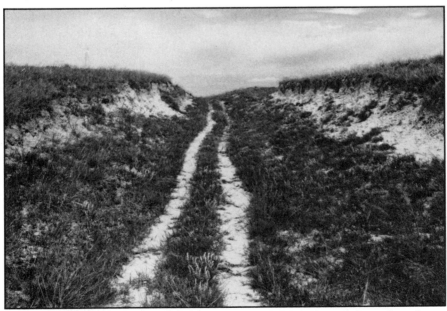

Wagon ruts cut deep into California Hill near Brule, Nebraska. Julie Fanselow photo.

crossed the Platte and started northwest, ultimately following the North Platte's course after a trek of about twenty-five miles across the high plains. The ford here was known as the "Lower California Crossing," taking its name because it was one of the two most popular crossings for those on their way to seek gold in California. (The other, used mostly after 1860, is the Upper California Crossing near Julesburg, Colorado, about thirty-five miles west.)

Continue west on Highway 30. About four miles west of town, watch for a historical marker on the right side of the road. It relates that California Hill now sits on land owned by the Oregon-California Trail Association, and that the site is dedicated to the memory of Irene D. Paden, who wrote *The Wake of the Prairie Schooner*, a vivid account of her own family's Oregon Trail explorations early in the 20th century. Malcolm Smith, a Paden fan from New York State, donated the money for the land purchase.

To reach the ruts, drive north up the dirt road about a half-mile. On the left, look for a white-paneled passageway through the barbed wire fence, thoughtfully erected in the summer of 1992 by the trails association. Park and walk through the gateway.

Start walking northwest past the windmill, looking for the Oregon Trail marker on the horizon. Keep an eye out for cattle—this is a grazing area—and for the occasional rattlesnake.

Unlike a lot of faint remnants along the Oregon Trail, there is no mistaking these ruts. The swale up the hill, started by wagon wheels, has been helped along by 150 years of erosion. Along this stretch, wood for fires was scarce. Tires popped off wagon wheels which had first expanded with the Platte's water, then shrunk in the dry air.

By the time the emigrants reached California Hill, they were about thirty-five days and 450 miles from Independence. More than three-quarters of their journey remained. They were tired, and this land was hot and windy, but they knew this was no place to turn back. If they had come this far, they could press on.

Modern-day visitors to this area will find it easy to understand what the emigrants endured. Yet from up on this rise, you also can see I-80, Highway 30, and the Union Pacific, with trains, trucks, and automobiles rushing east and west...proof once again that our nation's earliest transportation corridors usually proved to be the best.

From here, travelers can backtrack to Ogallala and take U.S. Highway 26 to Windlass Hill, or continue on the dirt roads, following the same general route of the Oregon Trail. In late spring or summer, two-wheel drives should stay on the highway due to the possibility of mud bogs on the back roads. But those traveling after Memorial Day or in a four-wheel drive vehicle should have no problem getting through the back way.

To do so, continue north to a corner, where you must turn left. Drive west for three miles, then north for four miles, then west again for two

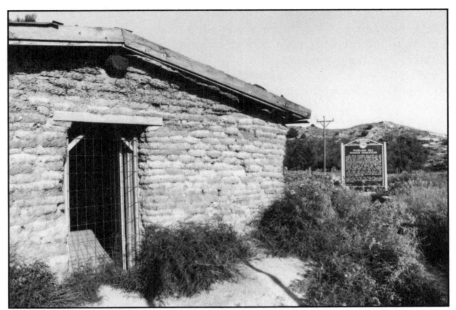

This sod house replica of a homesteader's cabin marks the entrance to Windlass Hill. Julie Fanselow photo.

more miles. (During this two-mile stretch, watch for the trail to intercept the road about 100 yards shy of the first mile intersection.) Turn north again; this road leads to Highway 26. Turn left at the highway intersection and proceed to Windlass Hill, about three miles to the west on the left.

WINDLASS HILL AND ASH HOLLOW

Judging from emigrant diaries, **Ash Hollow** was one of the most favored spots along the Oregon Trail. Here, the travelers found welcome shade trees and firewood, abundant grass for their animals, and water that one pioneer called "the best and purest ever drank...a beverage prepared by God himself." Indeed, many guidebooks pronounced the water at Ash Hollow the very best along the whole Oregon Trail. But before they could enjoy these treasures, the emigrants had to make their way down the dreaded **Windlass Hill**, the steepest descent yet encountered. Today, the incline offers a superb look at the power of natural forces over landscape, humans, and history.

Here, travelers tied ropes to their wagons, locked the wheels, and hoped for the best. One pioneer wrote that the drop was so terrifying that no one spoke the entire time; another noted that the hill was so steep that it seemed to hang "a little past the perpendicular." Diaries also told of broken wagons and broken bones among the animals and the emigrants themselves. Some travelers decided to avoid the hill altogether, keeping to the bluffs another sixteen or seventeen miles out of the way just to bypass the steep grade.

Despite the name "Windlass Hill," the pioneers apparently did not use windlasses (machines consisting of a cylinder wound with rope and turned by a crank) to ease the descent. A video at the Ash Hollow visitor center explains that such devices were never mentioned in emigrant diaries; if they were used at all, it must have been in later days.

To experience Windlass Hill, turn in the parking lot and walk up the path to a footbridge. Before crossing, note the deep scars that stretch off down the hill to the right. This was the Oregon Trail. Continue up the path to the top of the hill. Here, visitors can walk along the ruts a ways before returning to the crest of the hill, where today's travelers will see Windlass Hill as the emigrants saw it, steep and foreboding.

Before leaving the area, check out the sod house replica near the Windlass Hill entrance. The stones surrounding the historical marker near the house are all that remain of the original dwelling built in the late nineteenth century by Dennis B. Clary, a Methodist minister who was born in Maryland in 1822 and migrated to Nebraksa in 1885. Clary's humble home was reconstructed during the Ash Hollow Centennial Pageant in 1967.

Once they'd conquered Windlass Hill, the pioneers were free to frolic at Ash Hollow, which is actually a six-mile long plain stretching to the North Platte. Today, visitors can enjoy a picnic, watch the excellent video presentation at the visitor center, or stroll along a trail to either Ash Hollow Cave, used by prehistoric people as much as 6,000 years ago, or the site of Ash Hollow Spring.

Ash Hollow is interesting for reasons other than the Oregon Trail. Scientists have found evidence of prehistoric use dating back 7,000 to 10,000 years and of prehistoric animals including mammoths and mastodons. The area also figured prominently in the beginning of hostilities between Indians and whites. It was the site of a major battle between the Sioux and Pawnee in 1835. Later, eighty-six Sioux were killed during a 1855 battle with whites at nearby Blue Water Creek. Although Gen. Harney was initially hailed as a hero following this encounter, the battle later became known as the "Harney Massacre." The Blue Water Battle is considered one of the twelve largest engagements between Indians and whites in the United States, and it is the incident most often cited as precipitating the Indian Wars.

A Nebraska park permit is required for entry into Ash Hollow and Windlass Hill. Permits are available at the park office, which is open from 9 a.m. to 5 p.m. daily Memorial Day through Labor Day. Call (308) 778-5651 for more information.

A small cemetery on the left side of Highway 26 just past the Ash Hollow park exit is notable as the final resting place of Rachel E.

Pattison, who died June 19, 1849, at the age of eighteen. Like so many other emigrants, she woke up one morning in fine health, fell ill by noon, and was dead by sundown. The dreaded cholera had struck again, this time claiming a bride of just three months. Pattison's original headstone may still be seen encased behind glass at the grave.

Once past the cemetery, cross the Platte (the emigrants stayed on the river's south banks), and arrive in Lewellen, a small town with a few cafes and a gas station. Oshkosh, twelve miles west, has a bit more commerce, a couple of small museums, campgrounds, free swimming, and a nine-hole golf course.

Oshkosh also is home to Thunder Valley Western Excursions, a working ranch which offers two-hour Oregon Trail rides daily except Wednesdays from Memorial Day through Labor Day. Each participant is assigned an emigrant identity based on journal entries. The experience concludes with a steak dinner cooked over an open fire. Reservations are needed; for more information or to save a spot, call (308) 772-3906. The ranch is located two miles south of Oshkosh on Highway 27, then two miles west.

North of Oshkosh, Crescent Lake National Wildlife Refuge is popular for hiking, fishing, and bird watching. Past Oshkosh, it's a scenic fifty-minute drive along Highway 26 to Bridgeport, home of the trail's next major landmarks, Courthouse Rock and Jail Rock. As always, the North Platte River and the Union Pacific accompany the roadway. Nebraska Highway 92, which runs sixteen miles from Broadwater to Bridgeport, actually parallels the Oregon Trail more closely than does Highway 26.

COURTHOUSE ROCK AND JAIL ROCK

After several weeks on the Oregon Trail, the boredom could be intense. Emigrants sought to relieve it in a variety of ways: through music and dancing, card games, or conversation. But in what is now western Nebraska, the emigrants found a new source of entertainment in the strange, high rock formations that lined the route, serving as landmarks. Most of the pioneers were former Midwestern flatlanders, and they had never seen anything like these monolithic masses of stone.

Two of the best-known formations, **Courthouse Rock and Jail Rock**, are about five miles south of Bridgeport via Nebraska Highway 88. Although the Oregon Trail ran just south of what is now Bridgeport, few emigrants could resist the urge to trek south and see the formations up close. Or as Gregory Franzwa put it in *The Oregon Trail Revisited*, "After moving some 500 miles from Independence, another four miles was nothing, especially when it could be negotiated either on horseback or afoot, without wagons." Once they reached the rocks, many emigrants climbed them, which visitors can still do today.

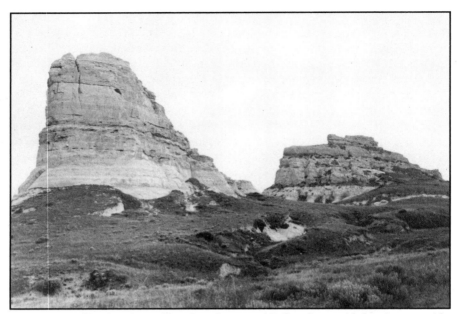

The naming of landmarks such as Courthouse and Jail rocks provided emigrants with a source of entertainment along the trail. Julie Fanselow photo.

As Franzwa also pointed out, Courthouse Rock (sometimes called Courthouse Block) may have gotten its name because it reminded emigrants of the courthouse in St. Louis, which at the time didn't yet have its tall, Italianate dome. Many pioneers probably carved their names on the sandstone and clay rocks, but these have long since worn away.

Enoch W. Conyers, who traveled the trail in 1852, had this to say as his party approached the area on June 16: "We came in view of Courthouse Block and Chimney Rock about noon today while crossing the ruins of the 'ancient bluffs.' We have a splendid view of those noted rocks from our camp tonight which brings to mind some verses composed by "The Platte River Poet,' one of which runs thus:

> 'The next we came to was Platte River
> Great sights were there to see.
> There was Courthouse Block and Chimney Rock
> And, next, Fort Laramie.'"

Courthouse and Jail rocks are at the eastern edge of a region known as the Wildcat Hills. Scenic Nebraska Highway 88 traverses the area, dead ending at Nebraska Highway 71. A right turn there leads past Wildcat Hills State Recreation Area and Game Reserve, where visitors can view buffalo, elk, and longhorn steer. People who visit in May or June may catch sight of a baby buffalo or elk, and coyotes and bobcats live in

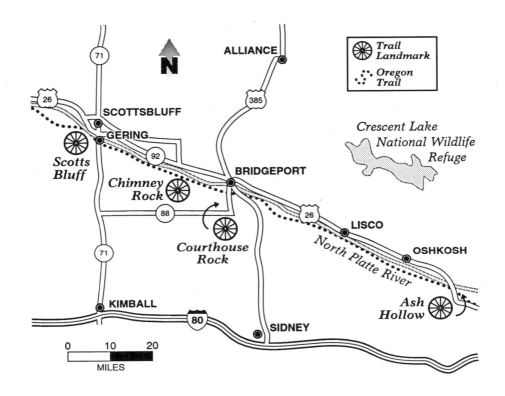

the area, too. The Wildcats offer abundant recreation and are popular with mountain bikers, campers, horseback riders, and hikers. Those who decide to take Highway 88 should first visit Chimney Rock, which is best accessed via Nebraska Highway 92. It's closer to Bridgeport than to Scottsbluff.

Bridgeport also was the home of Paul C. Henderson, who spent fifty-two years researching the emigrant trail. His grave in the cemetery west of town has been marked by the Oregon-California Trails Association. The Morrill County Fair takes place in Bridgeport in late August.

The area north of Bridgeport includes the Bridgeport State Recreation Area, just one mile north of town, and a most unusual roadside attraction thirty-eight miles north in Alliance. "Carhenge," featuring some thirty-five vehicles planted in the ground, is the Automobile Age's version of the mysterious Stonehenge monument near Salisbury, England. Alliance celebrates each year's summer solstice at the site with a parade, picnic, pageant, and bonfire. (No one should ever accuse Nebraskans of lacking a good sense of humor.) Bridgeport also is the jumping-off spot for the Black Hills and Badlands of South Dakota.

SIDEBAR: BLACK HILLS AND BADLANDS

Few areas of the West have as motley a mixture of natural and man-made attractions as does South Dakota's southwest corner. A three- to four-hour drive north of Bridgeport, Nebraska, will put travelers within reach of such sights as Mount Rushmore, Badlands and Wind Cave national parks, the world-famous Wall Drug, and the Pine Ridge Indian Reservation, one of the poorest and most storied in the United States.

Weed through the tourist traps and there's plenty to like about the region. Badlands National Park boasts a raw, rugged landscape and some of the world's finest fossil beds, formed about 37 million years ago during the Oligocene Epoch.

The Badlands offer backcountry adventure for those with time to explore. The Castle Trail is particularly acclaimed for its varied prairie topography and wealth of wildlife, including pronghorn antelope, bison, badgers, coyotes, and prairie dogs. Those in a hurry can drive the forty-mile loop road (South Dakota Highway 240) between Wall and Cactus Flat. Primitive camping is available, as are cabins at the Sioux-run Cedar Pass Lodge, located south of Cactus Flat. The White River Visitor Center, on the Pine Ridge Reservation in the park's South Unit, features displays and programs on Sioux history.

Wind Cave National Park, adjacent to Custer State Park on South Dakota Highway 87, offers daily subterranean tours during the summer. The excursions range from short candlelight walks to more strenuous spelunking expeditions. Jewel Cave National Monument, fourteen miles west of Custer, S.D., on U.S. Highway 16A, is one of the longest caves in the world. It too offers tours, as do a number of privately held caves scattered throughout the area.

The Black Hills were named by the Lakota Sioux for the dark appearance of their coniferous forests. The Sioux considered the land sacred, and their rights to it were ensured in a treaty signed in 1868. But the U.S. government broke the pact during the gold rush of the late 1870s. In recent years, the Supreme Court offered the Sioux $200 million as compensation for loss of their lands, but the Sioux are not interested. They want only the land, and their claim remains bogged down in the federal bureaucracy.

Today's Black Hills are heavily commercialized, but their beauty remains mostly intact. Check with the Forest Service office in Custer for maps and information on the area's many scenic byways (and for restrictions on motor homes and trailers, which may have trouble negotiating the region's roads).

Mount Rushmore is probably the best-known Black Hills attraction. Created under the direction of Gutzon Borglum, it features the sixty-foot-high heads of presidents George Washington, Thomas Jefferson, Abraham Lincoln, and Theodore Roosevelt. The sculpture is bathed in floodlights each night at dusk.

74

The Crazy Horse Memorial near Custer was started in 1947 by sculptor Korczak Ziolkowski to honor Chief Crazy Horse and the Native Americans. When completed, it will measure 563 feet high and 641 long, which would make it the largest statue in the world. It too is lit nightly at dusk.

Other Black Hills sights include Custer State Park, known for its eighteen-mile wildlife loop drive and abundant recreation, and Deadwood, which retains much of its old Wild West atmosphere (including small-stakes gambling). It was here that Wild Bill Hickok was shot in the back while playing poker in 1876. He's buried alongside Calamity Jane (who claimed she was his secret bride) in Mt. Moriah Cemetery overlooking the city.

Nearby, the town of Lead (ryhmes with greed) is famous for its Homestake Gold Mine, largest in the western hemisphere. And in early August, Sturgis attracts hordes of Harley enthusiasts for the Black Hills Motorcycle Classic. Spearfish is home to the Black Hills Passion Play, presented Sunday, Tuesday, and Thursday June through August. For more information on South Dakota, write the state Department of Tourism, Capital Lake Plaza, Pierre, SD 57501, or call (800) 843-1930 or (800) 952-2217 in South Dakota.

CHIMNEY ROCK

Of all the natural landmarks along the Oregon Trail, **Chimney Rock** is probably the most famous. Rising almost 500 feet above the North Platte River, Chimney Rock can be seen from thirty miles away. The emigrants watched it, entranced, for two to three days as their wagons rolled ever closer. Landmarks such as these eased the travelers' mind, for they could tell they were making progress. They could see for themselves that what they'd heard from friends and neighbors was true: the West was a strange and wondrous land, and the best was yet to come.

"At this place was a singular phenomenon, which is among the curiosities of the country," Captain Benjamin Bonneville wrote in 1832. "It is called the Chimney. The lower part is a conical mound rising up from the naked plain; from the summit shoots up a shaft or column, about one hundred and twenty feet in height, from which it derives its name."

Chimney Rock was a popular camping spot with good, dependable water. Thousands of pioneers climbed up the cone to carve their names, although these have long since worn away. There is no record, however, of anyone ever scaling the soft Brule clay spire, although some folks apparently tried—one emigrant noted a name etched in the chimney thirty feet up, and another may have died trying to beat that feat. There also are stories that some emigrants fired guns at the spire, claiming as souvenirs any chips they managed to knock off. And another story holds that in later years, the U.S. military used Chimney Rock for target practice. Even more recently, a lightning bolt zapped off a piece of the rock in 1972.

Every emigrant who kept a diary had something to say about Chimney Rock. Some gave it alternate nicknames: "lighting rod," "potato hill," and "beacon hill" were among the most descriptive. "The column that represents the chimney is crumbling away and fast disappearing," James Abbey wrote in 1850. In fact, the monument has probably eroded somewhat over the past 150 years, but not as much as the emigrants thought it would. In 1849, Joseph Hackney wrote that Chimney Rock was "the most remarkable object that I ever saw" and added that if it was situated in "the states," it would be visited by people from all over the world. Today, of course, it is.

For all its legendary and physical status, Chimney Rock stands pretty much on its own as a modern-day tourist attraction. Although it is a national historic site, the rock is interpreted only by a small, mobile visitor center along Nebraska Highway 92, which is open from 9 a.m. to 6 p.m. Memorial Day through Labor Day. The Nebraska State Historical Society Foundation has started a drive to raise nearly a half-million dol-

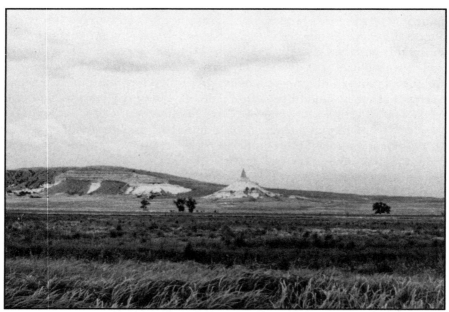

Chimney Rock is another distinct landmark along the trail in Nebraska. Julie Fanselow photo.

lars for a permanent visitor center, but it isn't certain when the center will be built.

To visit Chimney Rock up close, take the two-mile gravel road off Nebraska Highway 92. From a small parking lot a half-mile from the monument, it's a ten-minute walk to the base and another ten minutes or so up the cone. Sturdy footwear and long pants are advised, and hikers should watch out for rattlesnakes and thick brush.

Chimney Rock serves as backdrop for the Oregon Trail Wagon Train, a family-run tour company offering a variety of pioneer-style adventures. The nightly chuck wagon cookout includes a twenty-minute wagon ride and either stew or ribeye steak, followed by a campfire and songfest. Travelers who opt for the three-, four- or six-day wagon trips live much like the emigrants did. Activities on these trips include everything from prairie square dancing and muzzle loading instruction to Pony Express mail deliveries and artifact searches. Twenty-four-hour trips are available too, for those who think that one night without a soft bed and one morning without a shower is quite enough, thank you.

The Oregon Trail Wagon Train also offers Sunday-morning all-you-can-eat breakfasts, three-hour covered wagon tours to the Chimney Rock area, canoe rentals and shuttle service, campsites, and tours of a 1910 organic farm. Reservations are needed for all activities. Call (308) 586-1850 or write the Oregon Trail Wagon Train at P.O. Box 502, Bayard, NE 69334. The town of Bayard, just a few miles north of Chimney Rock, has one motel and a few restaurants and service stations. Its annual home-grown celebration, Chimney Rock Pioneer Days, takes place early in September with a Western art sale, parade, kidnappings by "outlaws," entertainment, and a pig roast.

From Chimney Rock, it's on to Scotts Bluff, another famous landmark, and Scottsbluff, western Nebraska's largest city. The town and the monument may be reached either by continuing west on Nebraska Highway 92, or by driving north through Bayard and west through Minatare on U.S. Highway 26. Minatare is near Lake Minatare State Recreation Area, home of some of the area's best camping and fishing. Lake Minatare also boasts Nebraska's only lighthouse, built between 1934 and 1936 by the Civilian Conservation Corps. The sixty-foot-high lighthouse can be ascended inside via a narrow spiral staircase.

SCOTTS BLUFF NATIONAL MONUMENT

One of the finest views on the Oregon Trail can be found atop **Scotts Bluff National Monument**. From here, visitors can see Chimney Rock and the Wildcat Hills to the east and even Wyoming's Laramie Peak, 120 miles to the west. This fortress-like landform is equally fascinating from the ground, looming over the twin towns of Scottsbluff and Gering like a "Nebraska Gibraltar."

Indians wandered through this area as much as 10,000 years ago, following the Platte to places where buffalo herds would stop to drink. Native peoples called the monolith "Me-a-pa-te," which meant "hill that is hard to go around." The first whites to see the bluff were probably a party of John Jacob Astor's men heading back East from the Pacific coast in 1812. Soon, the formation became a familiar sight to fur-traders and mountain men who traversed the North Platte route while heading to rendezvous and, later, trading posts in the Rockies and beyond.

The story goes that Hiram Scott was leading a trapping expedition through here in either 1828 or 1829 when he was left to die near Laramie Fork. The following spring, his remains were found at the base of Me-a-pa-te. Friends and fellow trappers recalled Scott's wish to someday be buried at the bluffs. How he got there is still a mystery, but the great Western landmark has been known as Scotts Bluff ever since.

Scotts Bluff offers an interesting geology lesson. Much of the monolith is being eroded away by wind and water, just as most of the surrounding Great Plains were worn down over the past fourteen million years. But Scotts Bluff is topped by an isolated patch of durable material known as "cap rock," which has served to protect the underlying sandstone, volcanic ash, and siltstone from the natural forces that have wiped out other nearby badlands.

Scotts Bluff so intimidated early wagon trains that they went well out of their way to avoid it, traveling through Robidoux Pass (named for a Missourian of French ancestry who set up several trading posts in the area) several miles to the south. Around 1850, the Mitchell Pass route through the bluff opened up and quickly gained favor. Mitchell Pass is right along present-day Highway 92; in fact, it is easily visible as you approach the monument from the east as the formidable gash that appears to split the bluff in two.

The monument visitor center is open from 8 a.m. to 5 p.m. daily. It has displays on the area's natural and human history, but the real highlight is the Oregon Trail Museum, which boasts the nation's best collection of photos, sketches, and paintings by William Henry Jackson, who first traveled west in 1866 after a broken engagement. A short trail leads to Jackson's campsite and to deep ruts left by emigrant wagons. Park rangers present Oregon Trail living history programs at Scotts Bluff each summer weekend. The visitor center also includes a very good selection of Oregon Trail interpretive material including maps, posters, slides, books, and post cards.

No Scotts Bluff visit would be complete without a trip to the top. A hike to the top and back takes about two hours, which allows time for explorations on the summit. Or drive up in minutes and spend time on the overlook trails. Watch for jack rabbits, rattlesnakes, prairie dogs, and assorted other little critters. The bird kingdom is represented by swifts, cliff swallows, magpies, and kestrels. It's important to stay on the trails to help prevent further erosion; rock along the Summit Trail is soft and

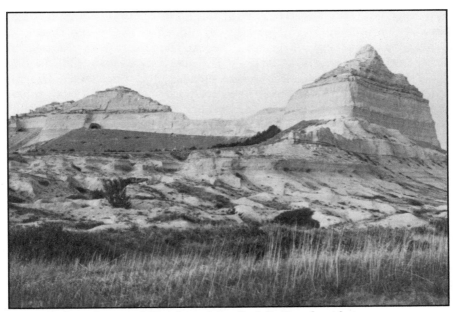
Scotts Bluff stands sentinel-like above the trail. Julie Fanselow photo.

crumbly, and leaving the trail could be dangerous. The Saddle Rock hiking trail is just over 1.5 miles long, one way. It includes some fairly steep sections and a few steps. Few emigrants had time to make the climb, but modern visitors should make every effort to do so. No one leaves disappointed.

The summit road is open from 8 a.m. to 4:30 p.m. Trailers are not permitted on the summit road, and the road may be closed in inclement weather. The park grounds are open from dawn to dusk all year. Admission to Scotts Bluff National Monument is $3 per car, good for a full seven days, and folks over 62 are admitted free. For more information, call (308) 436-4340.

If time is available, drive to **Robidoux Pass.** To get there, follow U.S. Highway 71 about 1.5 south miles past its intersection with U.S. Highway 92. Turn right on the gravel Robidoux Road.

Nine miles from the highway, watch for a historical marker on the left-hand side marking the supposed site of Robidoux's first trading post and blacksmith shop. Historians believe the site was actually across the gravel road a ways. Here, the Oregon Trail cut up the hillside on the left side of the modern road to avoid the deep arroyo. Several emigrant graves are also in the vicinity. Robidoux Pass is another 1.5 miles up the road, with the trail following on the right-hand side. At the pass is a commanding view of Laramie Peak. Turn around here and return to the highway or continue down the gravel road, which swings south then east through Carter Canyon. Leaving the canyon, the site of the second Robidoux Trading post is on the right. The road leads back to Highway 71.

Rebecca Winters was a Mormon pioneer who traveled the Oregon Trail with her family in 1852. They were on their way to Utah when cholera hit the wagon train somewhere west of Fort Kearny, and Rebecca died Aug. 15. She was buried and the grave was marked by an extra wagon tire on which a relative inscribed the words: "Rebecca Winters. Age 50." Years later, when laying a new route through the area, Burlington Railroad surveyors found the grave, still marked by the tire. The surveyors asked the railroad for permission to slightly alter the route to leave the grave undisturbed. Permission was granted, and the grave may still be seen.

To find it, turn east on Beltline Highway, which intersects with Highway 71 just north of the Platte River. Follow Beltline just over 2.25 miles southeast. Park at the electrical substation on the left-hand side of the road, and walk across the tracks to see the grave, which will be just a few paces west.

Those with any doubt that they're in the heart of Oregon Trail country can simply take a glance through the Scottsbluff/Gering phone book. Included are listings for the Oregon Trail Barber Shop, the Oregon Trail Church of the Nazarene, the Oregon Trail Eye Clinic, Oregon Trail Travel, Oregon Trail Hobbies, even Oregon Trail Plumbing, Heating, and Cooling. Each July, Gering holds its Oregon Trail Days bash. The event is one of Nebraska's oldest community celebrations, and it features an old settlers' reunion plus a parade, chili cook-off, athletic competitions, and big-name country entertainment.

There's still plenty to see and do for those who can't make it during mid-July. The North Platte Valley Museum at 11th and J in Gering has an eight-foot-square relief map of the various trails from Ogallala, Nebraska, to Douglas, Wyoming, as well as a fur trapper's bull boat, an 1895 sod house, and a settler's log cabin. The Wyo-Braska Museum of Natural History, also in Gering at 950 U Street, displays more than 200 mounted animals inside a renovated Union Pacific Depot. On a hot day, Gering's Oregon Trail Park is the place to be with its cool pool and 150-foot waterslide.

Scottsbluff is home to Riverside Park and Zoo, located at 1600 S. Beltline Highway West. An unusually large facility for a city of Scottsbluff's size, the zoo features lions, tigers, zebras, monkeys, mountain lions, leopards, and a river otter water slide. Special exhibits geared especially for kids include a prairie dog town, petting zoo, and playground.

Scottsbluff/Gering is the trade center of Nebraska's panhandle, so it offers plenty of choices for restaurants, lodging, and shopping, plus a little bit of nightlife: Check out the Oregon Trail Lounge on East Highway 92 in Gering for lively country music and dancing. Annual activities include summer repertory theater, the nation's second-largest antique-car race (the "Sugar Valley Rally," held early each June), the Scotts Bluff County Fair in mid-August, and a hot-air balloon festival in mid-October. For more information, contact the Scottsbluff/Gering United Chamber of Commerce at 1721 Broadway, Scottsbluff, NE 69363, or call (308) 632-2133.

From Scottsbluff, get back on U.S. Highway 26 and head west. Fort Laramie, the first major Oregon Trail attraction in Wyoming, is about an hour's drive away.

LODGING

FAIRBURY, NEBRASKA

Capri Motel, (402) 729-3317, Junction of Highways 136 and 15, $30-$55.

Holiday Motel, (402) 729-6151, West Highway 136, $25-$39.

Parker House Bed & Breakfast, (402) 729-5516, 515 1/2 Fourth St., $40-$55.

HEBRON, NEBRASKA

Rosewood Villa Motel, (402) 768-6524, 140 S. Highway 81, $40-$55.

Wayfarer Motel, (402) 768-7226, 104 N. 13th St. at Highway 81, $25-$40.

RED CLOUD, NEBRASKA

Green Acres Motel, (402) 746-2201, North Highway 281, $25-$40.

McFarland Hotel, (402) 746-3591, 141 W. 4th Ave.

Meadowlark Manor Bed & Breakfast, (402) 746-3550, 241 W. 9th Ave., $40-$55.

Richardson House Bed & Breakfast, (402) 746-3264, 202 N. Webster, $55 and up.

HASTINGS, NEBRASKA

Grand Motel, (402) 463-1369, 201 E. "J" St, $30-$40.

Holiday Inn, (800) 465-4329, 22nd St. and Highway 281 North, $55-$60.

Rainbow Motel, (402) 463-2989, 1000 W. "J" St., $31-$34.

X-L Motel, (800) 341-8000, 1400 W. "J" St., $31-$34.

GRAND ISLAND, NEBRASKA

Best Western Island Inn, (800)528-1234, 2311 S. Locust St., $30.

Conoco Motel, (308) 384-2700, 2107 W. 2nd St., $32.

Holiday Inn-Interstate 80, (800) 465-4329, I-80 Exit 312, $52.

Kirschke House Bed & Breakfast, (308) 381-6851, 1124 W. 3rd St., $55 and up.

Lazy V Motel, (800) 341-8000, 2703 E. Highway 30, $26.

Relax Inn, (308) 384-1000, 507 W. 2nd St., $30.

Riverside Inn, (308) 384-5150, 3333 Ramada Road, $40.

MINDEN, NEBRASKA

Pioneer Village Motel, (800) 445-4447, Highways 6, 34, and 10, $40-$44.

Prairie View Bed & Breakfast, (308) 832-0123, five miles east on Highway 74, $25-$40.

KEARNEY, NEBRASKA

Best Western Tel-Star, (800) 528-1234, 1010 3rd Ave., $51-$56.
Budget Host Western Inn, (800) 283-4678, 1401 2nd Ave., $38-$44.
Kearney Inn 4 Less, (308) 237-2671, 709 2nd Ave. E., $38.
Luxury Inn, (308) 234-5699, 619 2nd Ave. E., $38.
Pioneer Motel, (308) 237-3168, 917 E. 25th St at Highway 30, $25-$39.
Ramada Inn, (800) 228-2828, I-80 Exit 272, $64.
Super 8 of Kearney, (800) 843-1991, 15 W. 8th St.
Walden West Bed & Breakfast, (308) 237-7296, Fawn Woods Lake, $55 and up.

LEXINGTON, NEBRASKA

Best Western Minute Man Motel, (800) 528-1234, 801 S. Bridge St., $30-$34.
Econo Lodge, (800) 424-4777, I-80 Exit 237, $34.

COZAD, NEBRASKA

Best Western Circle S Motel, (800) 528-1234, 440 S. Meridian, $30.
Cozad Motel, (308) 784-2059, 712 Ave. K., $26.

GOTHENBURG, NEBRASKA

Travel Inn, (308) 537-3638, I-80 Exit 211, $25-$40.
Western Motor Inn, (308) 537-3622, I-80 Exit 211, $25-$40.

MAXWELL, NEBRASKA

Valley View Guest Ranch, (308) 582-4320, South of I-80 Exit 190.

NORTH PLATTE, NEBRASKA

Best Western Chalet Lodge, (800) 528-1234, 920 N. Jeffers St., $41-$45.
Budget Inn Park Motel, (308) 532-6834, 1302 N. Jeffers St., $26.
1st Interstate Inn, (308) 532-6980, I-80 Exit 177, $37.
Hilltop Bed & Breakfast, reservations at (402) 423-3480, $25-$40.
Motel 6, (308) 534-6200, I-80 Exit 177, $36.
Rambler Motel, (308) 532-9290, 1420 Rodeo Road, $23.
The Stockman Inn, (308) 534-3630, 1402 S. Jeffers St., $45-$53.
Travelers Inn, (800) 341-8000, 602 E. 4th St., $28-$32.

SUTHERLAND, NEBRASKA

Park Motel, (308) 386-4384, I-80 Exit 158.

PAXTON, NEBRASKA

Gingerbread Inn Bed & Breakfast, (308) 239-4265, I-80 Exit 145, $40-$55.

OGALLALA, NEBRASKA

Best Western Stagecoach Inn, (800) 528-1234, 201 Stagecoach, $55-$65.
1st Interstate Inn, (308) 284-2056, 108 Prospector Drive, $34-$40.
Holiday Inn, (800) 465-4329, 201 Chuckwagon Road, $47-$62.
Kingsley Lodge, (308) 284-2775, on Lake McConaughy, $40-$55.
North Shore Lodge, (308) 355-2222, on Lake McConaughy. Cabins.

OGALLALA, NEBRASKA (CONT.)

Oregon Trail Motel, (308) 284-3705, 214 E. 1st St.

Sunset Motel, (308) 284-4264, West Highway 30, $25-$40.

Super 8 Motel, (800) 843-1991, 500 E. "A" St. South, $40-$55.

OSHKOSH, NEBRASKA

S & S Motel, (308) 772-3350, Junction of Highways 26 and 27.

Shady Rest Motel, (308) 772-4115, Highway 26 and Main Street, $26.

BRIDGEPORT, NEBRASKA

Bell Motor Inn, (308) 262-0557, North Highway 385, $39.

Delux Motel, (308) 262-0290, 6th and Main streets.

Golden Acres Motel, (308) 262-0410, three miles north on Highway 385, $25-$40.

BAYARD, NEBRASKA

Landmark Inn, (308) 586-1375, 246 Main St., $26.

GERING, NEBRASKA

Cavalier Motel, (308) 635-3176, 3655 N. 10th St., $25-$40.

Circle S Lodge, (308) 436-2157, 400 "M" St., $40-$55.

SCOTTSBLUFF, NEBRASKA

Candlelight Inn, (800) 424-2305, 1822 E. 20th Place, $48-$52.

Capri Motel, (800) 642-2774, 2424 Ave. "I," $29-$33.

Comfort Inn, (800) 638-7949, 2018 Delta Drive, $43.

Lamplighter Motel, (800) 341-8000, 606 E. 27th St., $33.

Sands Motel, (308) 632-6191, 814 W. 27th St., $27-$29.

Scottsbluff Super 8, (800) 843-1991, 2202 Delta Drive.

The Scottsbluff Inn, (308) 635-3111, 1901 21st Ave., $44-$60.

Westward Ho Motel, (308) 632-6114, 1601 E, Overland Dr., $25-$40.

CAMPING

FAIRBURY, NEBRASKA

Rock Creek Station State Historical Park, (402) 729-5777, six miles southeast of town.

HEBRON, NEBRASKA

Hebron Riverside Park Campgrounds, 10th and Holdredge.

GRAND ISLAND, NEBRASKA

Mormon Island State Recreation Area, (308) 381-5649, I-80 Exit 312.

West Hamilton RV Park, (402) 886-2248, I-80 Exit 318 (Doniphan).

MINDEN, NEBRASKA

Pioneer Village Campground, (308) 832-2750, at Pioneer Village.

GIBBON, NEBRASKA

Windmill State Recreation Area, (308) 468-5700, I-80 Exit 285.

KEARNEY, NEBRASKA

Betty's I-80 RV Park, (308) 234-1072, I-80 Exit 263 (Odessa).

Clyde & Vi's Campground, (308) 234-1532, I-80 Exit 272.

Fort Kearny State Recreation Area, (308) 234-9513, adjacent to Fort Kearny State Historical Park.

LEXINGTON, NEBRASKA

Johnson Lake State Recreation Area, (308) 785-2685, seven miles south on Highway 283.

Masten's Camper Haven, (308) 324-3444, I-80 Exit 237.

GOTHENBURG, NEBRASKA

Lafayette Park, (308) 537-3867, one mile north of Highways 30 and 47.

Stage Stop Inn KOA, (800) 892-1947, I-80 Exit 211.

MAXWELL, NEBRASKA

Fort McPherson Campground, (308) 582-4320, two miles south of Exit 190, then half-mile west and half-mile south.

NORTH PLATTE, NEBRASKA

Holiday Trav-L-Park, (308) 534-2265, I-80 Exit 177, quarter-mile north, then half-mile east.

Lake Maloney State Recreation Area, (308) 532-6225, five miles south on Highway 83, then one mile west. Primitive sites.

OGALLALA, NEBRASKA

Lake McConaughy State Recreation Area, (308) 284-3542, nine miles north of Ogallala.

Lake Ogallala State Recreation Area, nine miles north of Ogallala.

Meyer Camper Court, (308) 284-2415, south of I-80 Exit 126.

Open Corral Camper Court, (308) 284-4327, I-80 Exit 126.

Van's Lakeview Fishing Camp, (308) 284-4965, on the south shore of Lake McConaughy at Gate 18.

BRULE, NEBRASKA

Riverside Campground, (308) 287-2474, I-80 Exit 117.

BRIDGEPORT, NEBRASKA

Bridgeport State Recreation Area, one mile north of town on U.S. Highway 26. Primitive sites.

Golden Acres RV Park, (308) 262-0410, three miles north on Highway 385.

GERING,NEBRASKA

Wildcat Hills State Recreation Area, (308) 436-2383, ten miles south on Highway 71. Primitive sites.

SCOTTSBLUFF, NEBRASKA

Lake Minatare State Recreation Area, (308) 783-2911, five miles east, then four miles north of Scottsbluff.

Riverside Park Campground, (308) 632-4136, southwest edge of city on Beltline Highway.

Scottsbluff/Chimney Rock KOA, (308) 635-3760, three-and-a-half miles west on Highway 26.

RESTAURANTS

FAIRBURY, NEBRASKA

The Courtyard Square, (402) 729-3388, 500 Fourth St. American cuisine. Salad and dessert bar at lunch.

Griffey's Restaurant & Lounge, (402) 729-9951, 400 Fourth St. Specializes in Nebraska beef and salads.

HEBRON, NEBRASKA

Ortman's Highway Cafe, Highway 81. Open 24 hours.

MINDEN, NEBRASKA

Pioneer Village Restaurant, (308) 832-1550, in Pioneer Village Motel. Casual dining, smorgasbord.

KEARNEY, NEBRASKA

Amigo's, (308) 237-2428, several locations including 4207 2nd Ave. Mexican food.

Captain's Table, (308) 237-5971, I-80 Exit 272 in the Ramada Inn. Seafood specialties.

Chef's Oven, (308) 236-6550. Adjacent to Best Western Tel-Star. Steaks, chicken, gourmet burgers, soups, and salads.

Gabby's Neighborhood Grill & Pub, (308) 236-8200, 3907 Central Ave.

The Lodge, (308) 234-2729, 1401 2nd Ave. Steak and seafood.

Tex's Cafe, (308) 234-3949, 23 E. 21st St.

Valentino's Ristorante, (308) 234-5545, 815 S. 2nd Ave. Italian food, pizza.

LEXINGTON, NEBRASKA

Little Paris Family Restaurant, (308) 324-5887, 201 E. 5th St. Home-cooked meals, salad bar, desserts.

GOTHENBURG, NEBRASKA

Bonnie's Swede Cafe, downtown Gothenburg. Homemade pies and rolls, Saturday night prime rib.

Homestead Restaurant, I-80 Exit 211. Salad bar, homemade cinnamon rolls, and pie.

Snack Shack, 516 Lake. Hamburgers, homemade pies.

NORTH PLATTE, NEBRASKA

The Airport Inn, (308) 534-4340, at Lee Bird Field. Breakfast, lunch and dinner at the airport.

Brick Wall, (308) 532-7545, 507 N. Dewey. Dining amid antique displays.

Fireplace Dining Room, (308) 534-3630, 1402 S. Jeffers St. In the Stockman Inn.

NORTH PLATTE, NEBRASKA (CONT.)

Golden Corral, (308) 534-3359, 901 S. Dewey. Steaks, seafood, large salad bar.

Hunan Chinese Restaurant, (308) 532-8145, I-80 and Highway 83 in the Nebraskan Motel. Mandarin, Hunan, Szechuan, and Cantonese cuisine.

PAXTON, NEBRASKA

Ole's Big Game Lounge & Grill, (308) 239-7500, I-80 Exit 145. Steaks, seafood, chicken, buffalo burgers. More than 200 big-game trophies on display.

OGALLALA, NEBRASKA

Front Street Steakhouse, (308) 284-4601, Downtown on Highway 30. Steaks, salad bar, kids' menu.

Hill Top Inn, (308) 284-4534, at Kingsley Dam nine miles north of Ogallala. Scenic view of Lake McConaughy, daily specials.

Hokes Cafe, (308) 284-4654, 302 E. 1st. Home cooking featuring chicken fried steak, fried chicken, steaks.

The Paddock Restaurant, (308) 284-3656, in the Best Western Stagecoach Inn. Sunday champagne brunch, weekly ethnic specialties.

Peking Chinese Restaurant, (308) 284-8300, 112 E. "A" St. Szechuan, Peking and Cantonese cuisine.

Pioneer Trails Restaurant, (308) 284-2388, in Pioneer Trails Mall (55 River Road). Informal dining featuring steaks and prime rib (Wednesdays and Saturdays).

BRIDGEPORT, NEBRASKA

Bell Restaurant, (308) 262-0557, north on Highway 385 in Bell Motor Inn. Informal dining featuring steaks.

SCOTTSBLUFF, NEBRASKA

Bush's Gaslight Restaurant & Lounge, (308) 632-7315, 2929 N. 10th. Casual dining. Steaks, seafood, chicken.

Country Kitchen, (308) 635-3800, 3605 N. 10th. Open 24 hours.

Grampy's Pancake House & Restaurant, (308) 632-6906, 1802 E. 20th Place. Large menu, breakfast served anytime.

Henry's Restaurant, (308) 635-7646, 1901 21st Ave. in the Scottsbluff Inn.

Oriental House, (308) 632-3922, 1502 E. 20th. Chinese cuisine. Closed Sundays.

Rosita's Restaurant, (308) 632-2429, 1205 E. Overland. Mexican food.

Vi's Diner, (308) 632-4000, 2223 Broadway. Daily buffets.

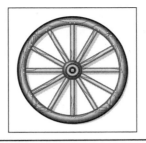

CHAPTER FIVE

HALFWAY TO HEAVEN: WYOMING

"We have crossed the great divide...the valley or gateway is ten to twenty miles wide...the ascent so gradual that we were scarcely aware that the culmination was reached and passed."
—Emigrant David R. Leeper at South Pass, 1849

FORT LARAMIE

It's tempting to think of the Oregon Trail as a lonely route, with a few huddled wagons traveling together across the vast, empty plains. But during the peak years of travel, the trail was in fact quite crowded, with one wagon company after another rolling westward. Nowhere was the congestion more evident than near the six major forts along the route.

The forts were crucibles of humanity, full of emigrants from the Midwest mingling with fur traders, military men, trappers, and Indians. Here the pioneers gathered to rest, repair their wagons, replenish supplies, and swap advice and stories with their fellow travelers. Until Fort Kearny was built in 1848, **Fort Laramie** was the first such outpost along the Oregon Trail.

Fort Laramie—then known as Fort William—was built by fur trader William Sublette in 1834. He sent word to the nearby Sioux and Chey-

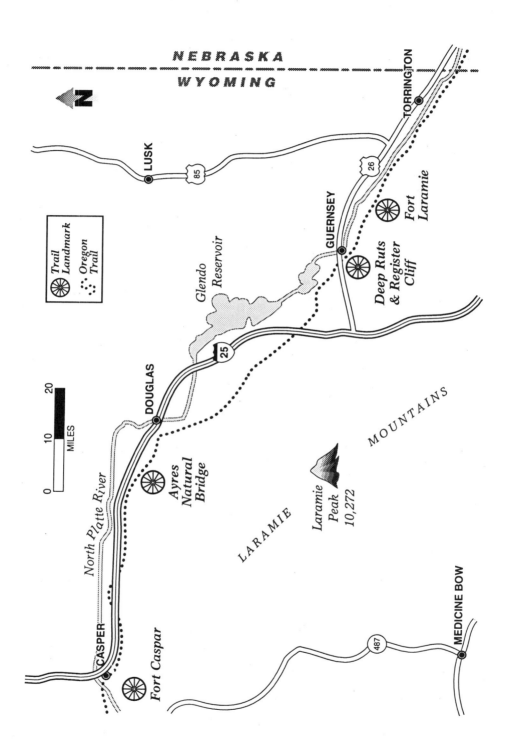

NEBRASKA

WYOMING

N

LUSK
85

TORRINGTON

26

GUERNSEY

Fort
Laramie

Deep Ruts
& Register
Cliff

Glendo
Reservoir

Trail
Landmark
Oregon
Trail

25

DOUGLAS

20

10

MILES

0

North Platte River

Ayres
Natural
Bridge

MOUNTAINS

Laramie
Peak
10,272

LARAMIE

CASPER

Fort Caspar

487

MEDICINE BOW

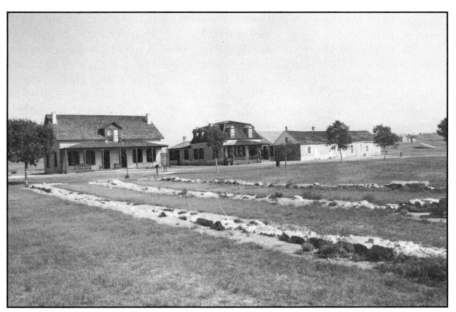

The officers' quarters are some of the remains of old Fort Laramie, Wyoming. Julie Fanselow photo.

enne chiefs that he wished to do business with them, but it wasn't until the American Fur Company bought the post two years later that it became a major trading post—at least until 1841, when a competing post, Fort Platte, was built just a mile away. The American Fur Company responded by replacing the rotting, wooden Fort William with a larger adobe structure they then named Fort John. Later, the fort became known as Fort Laramie after an obscure French-Canadian trapper, Jacques LaRamee, who may have been the first white man to see the area. Despite his low profile, LaRamee ended up giving his name to many of the most prominent features in eastern Wyoming, including Laramie Peak, the Laramie River, and the city of Laramie.

Fort Laramie was always a popular stop along the trail. But as emigrant traffic increased, relations between the whites and the Indians deteriorated rapidly, leading to calls for protection. The Army bought the post in 1849 and converted it to a military outpost. After Oregon Trail traffic trickled off in the 1860s, the site became a major staging area for campaigns against the Indians and later, as a buffer between whites and the few Indians who refused to submit to life on the reservations. It also served as a stopping place for prospectors on their way to the gold fields of South Dakota's Black Hills. Finally, with the end of Indian hostilities, the Army abandoned the post in 1890.

Fort Laramie is now a National Historic Site run by the National Park Service. It is located three miles southwest of the town of Fort Laramie ("250 Good People and Six Sore Heads," the sign says) off Highway 26. Begin with a stop in the visitor center, located in the old Commissary Storehouse. Here are exhibits on the fort's history and three thirty-minute videos: "Red Sunday," on the Battle of the Little Big Horn; "A Day in the Life of Fort Laramie;" and "The Oregon Trail." The center's bookstore has an excellent selection of books, maps, posters, and emigrant diaries from the Oregon Trail.

Children ages 6 through 12 are invited to take part in Fort Laramie's "Junior Ranger" program by asking for an activity packet at the visitor center before touring the fort. Living history programs take place daily from 9:30 a.m. to 5 p.m. during the summer, and people dressed in period costume present information on such places as the trader's store, bakery, calvary barracks, laundry, officer's quarters, and the guardhouse. Other special annual events include an Old-Fashioned Fourth of July, moonlight tours, old-time fiddlers, and Native American Heritage Days.

During the summer, thirty-minute interpretive talks on a variety of a topics are scheduled at 10 a.m., 11:30 a.m., and 2 p.m. daily. Ask at the visitor center for program topics and locations. One-hour ranger-led tours are offered at 10:30 a.m., 1 p.m., and 3 p.m. between June 15 and Aug. 15. Meet at the south end of the calvary barracks. Visitors can also tour the fort with the self-guiding brochure available at the visitor center.

Several sites are of special interest. Old Bedlam, built in 1849, housed bachelor officers and is the oldest military building in Wyoming. The structure was almost ninety years old and near collapse when the federal government re-acquired it and started a stabilization and reconstruction program. The hospital ruins were built on the site of an old Army cemetery used until 1868. The site of the original Fort John may be seen on the banks of the Laramie River behind the Captain's Quarters.

Travelers can take a break after their tour with a root beer, apple cider, or sarsaparilla at the Enlisted Men's Bar, located at the Post Trader's Store, or with a picnic on the grounds near the parking lot. There is no food, lodging, or camping at Fort Laramie, but all are available in nearby towns. Fort Laramie National Historic Site is open from 8 a.m. to 4:30 p.m. every day except Thanksgiving, Christmas, and New Year's Day, with extended hours from early June through Labor Day. Admission is $1 for people over 16; anyone under that age is admitted free. For more information, call (307) 837-2221.

Return to Highway 26 and continue driving west. It's only thirteen miles to Guernsey, home to Register Cliff and some of the best ruts on the Oregon Trail.

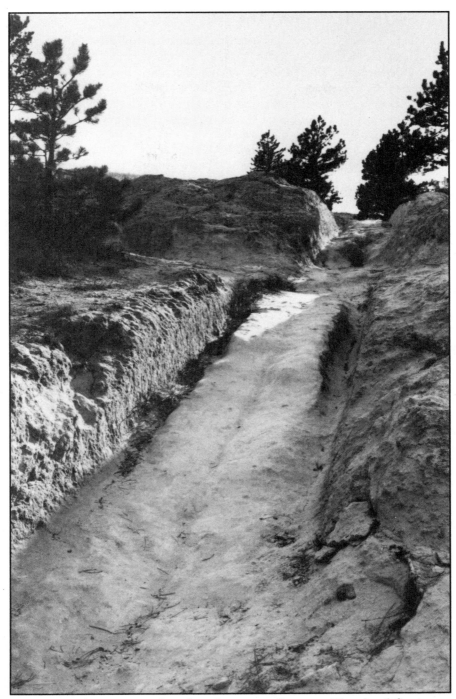

The passage of wagons over the soft sandstone near Guernsey, Wyoming, left ruts nearly five feet deep. Photo courtesy of the Wyoming Division of Tourism.

REGISTER CLIFF AND THE GUERNSEY RUTS

Just east of Guernsey, a Wyoming state rest stop offers a panoramic viewing area where visitors can look through a series of posts drilled with peepholes at landmarks including Mexican Hill, which emigrants traversed to regain the Platte River route after visiting Fort Laramie; Sand Point, a popular pioneer campsite; and Laramie Peak, which was the travelers' first evidence that they'd successfully crossed the high plains and made it to the mountains.

Once you reach Guernsey, follow the signs through town to **Register Cliff.** This popular campsite was about a day's travel west of Fort Laramie, and the sandstone cliff is covered with the names of people who passed through the area en route to Oregon or other points west. Unfortunately, many of the old signatures have either eroded away or been covered by those of more recent vintage. A good number of names from the 19th century are still visible, however, especially behind the fenced area that begins about 150 feet from the parking lot. Trail remnants can also be seen at Register Cliff, as can the graves of several unknown pioneers.

Alva Unthank of Wayne County, Indiana, traveled the trail in 1850 and was one of the many emigrants who signed his name on the cliff. He didn't last much longer; his grave, dated July 2, 1850, can still be seen

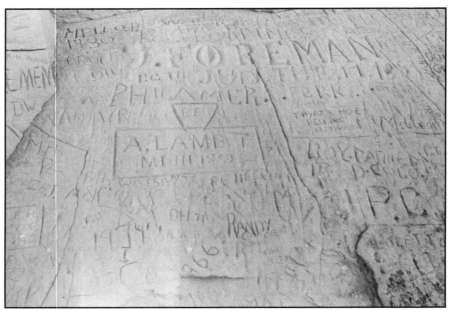

Register Cliff is covered with names of people who traveled through Wyoming along the Oregon Trail. Julie Fanselow photo.

near Glenrock. Historians believe he died of cholera or dysentery. In later years, Unthank's nephew, O.N. Unthank, and great-grandson, O.B. Unthank, added their names. Gregory Franzwa reported in *The Oregon Trail Revisited* that the names could still be found about thirty yards past the stone monument at Register Cliff, but this author was unable to locate them in the summer of 1992.

From Register Cliff, return to the road and head back toward Guernsey, but turn left into the **Oregon Trail Ruts State Historic Site.** Park and climb the 400-foot trail to the ruts. Many trail remnants along the Oregon Trail are faint or visible only to those with active imaginations. Not so here. Rugged terrain forced the wagons to travel across a narrow ridge of sandstone, wearing ruts that are up to five feet deep in some places! These are probably the most famous ruts along the entire Oregon Trail. When leaving the site, note the grave of Lucinda Rollins, who died here in June 1849. A white monument marks the grave, just across the road from the ruts parking area and slightly to the west.

Guernsey is home to the Wyoming Army National Guard, which means visitors to Register Cliff and the trail ruts must often contend with soldiers loudly conducting air maneuvers in the clear blue Wyoming sky overhead. But the town also claims Guernsey State Park, a popular recreation area that offers camping, Volksmarch programs and other hiking opportunities, picnicking, water sports, and a museum. Bluffs surrounding the reservoir block the wind, creating scenic campgrounds and prime conditions for boating and swimming—but not for sailboating or sailboarding. For that, try Glendo State Park about thirty-five miles northwest via I-15. Some Wyoming state parks charge entrance fees, which in 1992 were $3 for out-of-state vehicles and $2 for vehicles with Wyoming plates.

AYRES NATURAL BRIDGE

One of the prettiest spots near the emigrant route, **Ayres Natural Bridge** actually sits about a mile south of the Oregon Trail. But it's no wonder travelers went out of their way to see it. The site was donated to Converse County, Wyoming, by Andrew Clement Ayres in May 1920, and the county has preserved it as a pleasant park. (Some maps and guidebooks refer to the site as Ayers Natural Bridge; Wyoming highway department signs on I-25, shying from the spelling dispute, simply call it "Natural Bridge.")

LaPrele Creek is responsible for nature's handiwork at Ayres Natural Bridge. Over time, the creek wore its way through a sandstone monolith, carving a passageway and creating one of Wyoming's earliest tourist attractions. Ayres remains the only natural bridge with a stream running under it in the United States, and red rock formations and leafy shade trees add to the park's overall beauty.

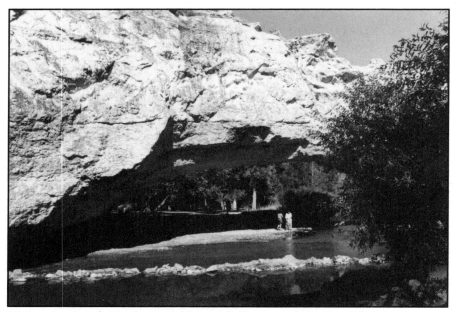

Visitors are dwarfed by the Ayres Natural Bridge west of Douglas, Wyoming. Julie Fanselow photo.

Activities at the park range from picnicking to fishing and hiking. Campers are welcome too, and a small grassy area set aside for tents looks particularly pleasant. The park is open for day use from 8 a.m. to 8 p.m. April 1 through Oct. 31, and admission is free. To get there, take the Natural Bridge exit off of I-25 eleven miles west of Douglas, then follow the signs five miles south to the park. The access road's last stretch may be too winding and steep for vehicles towing trailers.

Douglas, Wyoming, was founded in 1886 as a supply post for cattlemen and a rail distribution point. Today, it serves as home to 5,100 people and as world capital of the jackalope, a uniquely Western mix of jackrabbit, pronghorn antelope, and frontier fable. Specimens are available on every post card rack and in many bars in Wyoming, and skeptics can see a ten-foot replica at Third and Center streets in Douglas. The Converse County seat is also home to the Wyoming State Fair, held every third week in August since 1905, and to the Wyoming Pioneer Museum, located at the state fairgrounds.

In addition to these in-town activities, Douglas is at the hub of a wide range of outdoor attractions. Medicine Bow National Forest begins south of town and sprawls out across 1,665,755 acres in southeast Wyoming. The Douglas District includes Laramie Peak and the rest of the rugged Laramie Mountains. To the north, Thunder Basin National Grassland was turned into a dustbowl by homesteaders who used farming techniques more suited to wet climates. Today, the reclaimed 1.8 million-acre grassland is used primarily for grazing and energy resources development.

Even farther north is Devil's Tower National Monument, which is definitely worth a visit for those with an extra day. The stump-shaped rock monolith rises 867 feet from the ground and was proclaimed the first U.S. national monument in 1906 by President Theodore Roosevelt. Today, it is enjoyed by campers and climbers, and the nearby Belle Fourche River offers good fishing, swimming, and tubing opportunities. A prairie dog town rounds out the attractions at this fascinating site. Devil's Tower is twenty-eight miles northwest of Sundance via Wyoming Highway 24, about 190 miles from Douglas.

At least five dude ranches in the Douglas area offer genuine Western experiences to willing city slickers. For information, contact the Wagonhound Ranch, 1061 Poison Lake Road, Douglas, WY 82633, (307) 358-5439; Pellatz Ranch, 1031 Steinle Road, Route 2, Douglas, (307) 358-2380; Deer Forks Ranch, Route 6, 1200 Poison Lake Road, Douglas, (307) 358-2033; 09 Angus Ranch, 1681 Esterbrook Road, Douglas, (307) 358-2605; or Two Creek Ranch, 800 Esterbrook Road, Douglas, (307) 358-3467.

After leaving Ayres Natural Bridge and returning to Interstate 25, it's less than an hour's drive to Casper, one of Wyoming's largest cities and the home of Fort Caspar, another major post along the Oregon Trail.

SIDETRIP: INDIAN SITES IN NORTHEAST WYOMING

The opening of the Oregon Trail had a profound effect on white American history, but it had an equally large impact on the lives of the North American Indians. For centuries, tribes had lived basically simple lives close to the land of the plains and mountains of the West. When the whites' emigration began, relations between the cultures were mostly cordial. But increased traffic on the paths the Indians pioneered eventually led to misunderstandings, conflict and violence.

Northeast Wyoming has a high concentration of sites that trace the clash between the Indians and whites. One of the earliest events—and one tied directly to the Oregon Trail—was the Grattan Massacre, which took place near present-day Lingle. In August 1854, a Mormon wagon train traveling along the route to Oregon camped ten miles below Fort Laramie. After a stray cow belonging to the Mormons was killed by an Indian, a group of twenty-nine soldiers led by 2nd Lt. John Grattan was dispatched to the Indian camp to arrest the guilty man. The ensuing fight resulted in the deaths of Grattan and half his men, as well as an Indian chief. But even more crucially, the fight marked the start of years of intermittent hostilities along the trail. A monument to the incident stands three miles west of Lingle on Wyoming Highway 157. The U.S. soldiers who died were first buried on the battlefield then later removed to Fort McPherson National Cemetery back in Nebraska.

Fort Fetterman, eleven miles northwest of Douglas on Wyoming Highway 93, was located near the intersection of the Oregon and Bozeman trails. The Indians hated the "Bloody" Bozeman Trail, for it cut across their hunting grounds to the gold fields of Montana. The fort was established in 1867 and rapidly became a major supply post during U.S. military campaigns against the Indians. It is now a state-run historic site where the restored officers' quarters and ordnance building may be seen. A museum displays weapons, clothing, and artifacts from the period.

Some of the most famous events of the 1860s occurred near Fort Phil Kearny, which is about 145 miles north of Casper (take Exit 44 off of Interstate 90 north of Buffalo, Wyoming). Battles involving such famous Indians as Red Cloud and Crazy Horse were fought nearby, and exhibits at the fort museum help explain the events, which included the Fetterman Massacre of William Fetterman and his eighty-two men in 1866 and the Wagon Box Fight, in which soldiers shielded by wagon boxes and backed by new Springfield breech-loaded rifles survived a Sioux assault in 1867. The actual sites of these battles are within three miles of Fort Phil Kearny.

Those interested in the West's military history might want to keep driving north on I-90 into Montana and the site of the Battle of the Little Bighorn. Here, Lt. Col. George A. Custer and the 210 men of the Seventh Cavalry Regiment made their last stand against the Sioux and Northern Cheyenne in 1876. The main entrance is via Exit 510 on I-90, about seventy miles north of Sheridan, Wyoming. Tours are available. For more information on these sites, call Fort Fetterman at (307) 358-2864, Fort Phil Kearny at (307) 684-7629, or the Little Bighorn Battlefield National Monument at (406) 638-2621.

FORT CASPAR

For more than 400 miles—past Chimney Rock, Scotts Bluff, and Fort Laramie—the emigrants had traveled within sight of the Platte River. Now, they were about to leave it behind for the final dusty approach to South Pass, where they'd enter the Oregon Territory.

Some emigrants crossed the North Platte at the site of present-day Casper and took the northern route through Emigrant Gap and past Poison Spring, where pristine ruts still exist. Others waited a few more miles and made the ford upstream at Bessemer Bend. In either case, the North Platte crossing marked the beginning of some miserable travel, with good water and good grazing in very short supply. **Fort Caspar** was established to protect the emigrants as they made this important move.

The pioneers got across the North Platte in a variety of ways. Until 1847, they had to either improvise a ferry or hope for low water at the usual ford, four miles northeast of Fort Caspar. In 1847, Mormon leader Brigham Young established a ferry across the river and charged four to five dollars per wagon. When he founded the ferry, Young was on his way to establish the Mormon community near the Great Salt Lake. He left nine men behind to the operate the ferry, which helped raise money for the Mormon's new stronghold. The ferry stayed in operation through 1851.

Sometimes emigrants balked at either the fee or the time spent waiting to use the Mormon Ferry and tried to make their own crossing, even in high water. Emigrant James A. Pritchard wrote of one such instance in 1849, when his wagon train arrived on a Sunday and found 175 wagons already waiting to use the ferry: "We however joined another company or two and constructed a raft to cross our wagons on. After several efforts we succeeded in crossing two wagons, but we found the current so strong and the raft so heavy and unwieldy that we abandoned the project and awaited our turn which came in on Wednesday morning."

In 1852, John Richard—or Reshaw, as he was better known—built a wooden toll bridge over the North Platte at what is now Evansville, Wyoming, three miles from Casper. Reshaw's bridge served the emigration

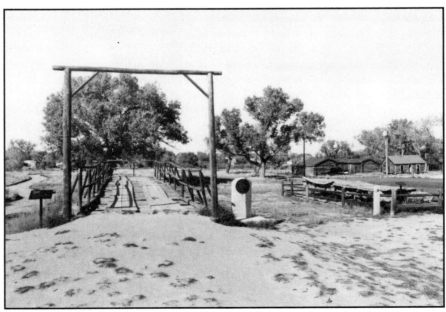

The Guinard Bridge and the Mormon Ferry have been reconstucted at Fort Caspar. Julie Fanselow photo.

off and on until 1865, and some historians say it put the Mormon Ferry out of business. In later years, however, Reshaw had competition from a 1,000-foot log bridge built in 1858 at the site of the Mormon Ferry by Louis Guinard.

Guinard charged a toll of $1 to $6, depending on river conditions. His bridge was used until 1867, when it was burned by Indians after the abandonment of Fort Caspar. Guinard also established a trading post at the site, and it became known as Platte Bridge Station. Later, the site was renamed in honor of Lt. Caspar Collins, who was killed while protecting a supply train from Indian attack in 1865.

As a military post, Fort Caspar played a key role in protecting the emigration as it moved up the Sweetwater Valley. It also helped preserve communications during the era by protecting a Pacific Telegraph office built at the south end of Guinard's bridge. Today, the reconstructed fort is the centerpiece of a popular Casper park. (An early recorder's spelling error accounts for the discrepancy between the name of the fort and the city that followed.)

Start a visit to Fort Caspar with a stop in its museum, which explains the history of the area and other Wyoming lore. Visitors can also pick up brochures for a self-guided tour of the reconstructed fort, which includes a sutler's store, blacksmith shop, officers' quarters, and several other buildings. Another self-guided trail combines nature and history, making its way past the piled earth and rock on which Guinard's bridge rested, the Oregon Trail itself, and "The Sand Bar," an infamous district well known in Casper's early days for its gambling and prostitution. The area was cleaned up in the 1940s, but a small white house—once a bordello—was saved as evidence of the former red-light district.

Fort Caspar is the site of several annual special events, including a mountain man rendezvous, Civil War encampment, lecture series, and Christmas candlelight tours. The complex also includes Centennial Park, where kids can have a ball on the playground.

To get to Fort Caspar, take the Poplar Street exit off of Interstate 25, turn left, then follow the signs to the fort, located on the west outskirts of town near the fairgrounds. The fort is open during the summer, and the museum is open year-round. Winter hours are from 9 a.m. to 5 p.m. weekdays and 1 to 4 p.m. Sundays, while the summer schedule is from 9 a.m. to 6 p.m. weekdays, 9 a.m. to 5 p.m. Saturdays and noon to 5 p.m. Sundays. Admission is free. For more information, call (307) 235-8462.

After visiting Fort Caspar, take a right on Wyoming Boulevard and proceed south to CY Avenue, which turns into Wyoming Highway 220, the main route to Bessemer Bend and Independence Rock.

SIDETRIP: URBAN WYOMING

With not quite a half a million residents—fewer than five per square mile—Wyoming ranks dead last among the fifty states in population. But even Wyoming has its pockets of city life.

Although emigrant trail commerce and cattle ranching were Casper's earliest industries, the town really took off in 1889 when the first oil well was tapped. From that modest beginning, Casper grew into the hub of the Rocky Mountain oil-and-gas industry. The boom created prosperity, and scandal too: In 1927, U.S. Secretary of the Interior Albert Fall went to prison for secretly leasing the nearby Teapot Dome oil field to the Mammoth Crude Co. without seeking bids from other companies.

In Wyoming's early days, Casper and Cheyenne vied to be the state's capital. The rivalry continues today as the two towns see-saw in their bids to be Wyoming's largest city. In the 1980 Census, Casper was larger; by 1990, Cheyenne had taken the lead. (Each town's population fluctuates between 45,000 and 50,000.)

But Casper has class. The Nicolaysen Art Museum at 400 E. Collins Dr. is housed in a refurbished warehouse and includes permanent and traveling exhibitions of major regional and national artists. The Discovery Center, a children's museum, is on the same site. The Casper Municipal Band plays each Thursday evening in Washington Park on McKinley Street, and several other groups showcase local dramatic, musical, and artistic talent. Rockhounds may want to visit the Tate Museum, open weekdays on the Casper College campus. The Werner Wildlife Museum at 405 E. 15th St. is another popular attraction.

Casper's biggest annual event is the Central Wyoming Fair and Rodeo, held the last week of July. Recreational opportunities include the Casper Recreation Center at 1801 E. Fourth St. and the Casper Family YMCA at 315 E. 15th. Both offer daily passes. Visitors can also take advantage of four city pools or the Casper Community Golf Course, at 2120 Allendale Blvd. Casper Mountain and Edness K. Wilkins State Park, both south of town, cater to outdoor fun and adventure. For shopping, try downtown or the Eastridge Mall, located at East Second and Wyoming Boulevard off of I-25.

Cheyenne's claim to fame is Frontier Days. The main attraction is the world's oldest and largest rodeo, also known as the "Daddy of 'em All," but free pancake breakfasts (with the batter mixed by cement truck) and the overall party-hearty atmosphere keep everyone happy, no matter what their interests. Be forewarned that Cheyenne motel prices double during Frontier Days, so plan accordingly.

Year-round, visitors to Cheyenne enjoy the Wyoming State Museum, 2301 Central Ave., and the Cheyenne Frontier Days Old West Museum at Eighth and Carey streets. The Cheyenne Club at 1617 Capitol Ave. features live country entertainment, and the Old Atlas Theater at 211 W. 16th St. offers vaudeville-style melodramas each summer. The state capitol is open to visitors from 8:30 a.m. to 4:30 p.m. weekdays, and tours are available. Frontier Mall, with seventy-five stores on Dell Range Boulevard, is Cheyenne's largest shopping center.

As home of the state's only four-year institution of higher learning, Laramie ranks as Wyoming's intellectual and cultural capital. The University of Wyoming holds a Western music festival each June, along with other arts activities year-round. But this is still Wyoming, and outdoor activities reign supreme. Popular spots include Curt Gowdy State Park (named for the sportscaster, a native Wyomingite) and Vedauwoo, both southeast of Laramie via I-80. Vedauwoo is one of North America's finest rock-climbing sites. In the summer, consider a scenic drive over the 10,847-foot Snowy Range Pass highway between Rawlins and Laramie.

For more information, contact the chambers of commerce in Casper (800-852-1889), Cheyenne (800-426-5009), or Laramie (307-745-7339).

BESSEMER BEND AND THE RED BUTTES

Not everyone had the time or money to use the ferry or toll bridge at present-day Casper. Many parties continued along the Platte to **Bessemer Bend**, the last place they could cross, and the site of an early U.S. Mail station after 1848. Today, Bessemer Bend is marked with a Bureau of Land Management interpretive shelter and by nature itself—the Red Buttes that served as a landmark to Indians, fur traders, and emigrants may still be seen south of the river.

Bessemer Bend was a popular campsite, used as early as 1812 by Robert Stuart and the Astorians, who were returning to St. Louis from the Pacific. From here, the route west to the Sweetwater River involved three days of rough, dry country and poisonous alkali water. John Fremont, passing through in 1842, commented on "innumerable quantities of grasshoppers," which had destroyed the grass. Today, Bessemer Bend is a popular put-in for floating downriver to Casper, a seven-mile trip. Picnic tables are available.

To get to Bessemer Bend, take Highway 220 six miles south of Casper. Turn right on the Bessemer Bend Road and continue three miles.

From here, Oregon Trail explorers have two choices. Stay on Highway 220, or follow the pioneers' route more closely by taking a forty-mile trip along back roads that meet Highway 220 just north of Independence Rock. The dirt-road alternative includes such trail landmarks as Emigrant Gap, Avenue of Rock, Willow Spring, and Poison Spring, but the way is not well marked. For exact directions and road conditions, inquire locally at Fort Caspar (235-8462), the Casper Chamber of Commerce (234-5311), or the Casper BLM district office (261-7600).

Travelers who stay on Highway 220 will glimpse several sweeping vistas of Alcova and Pathfinder reservoirs. Boating, fishing, and camping are all enjoyed along the shores of these great lakes. The BLM maintains

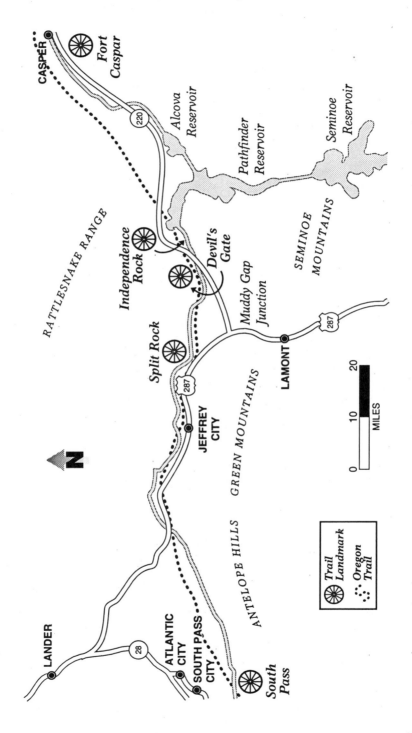

101

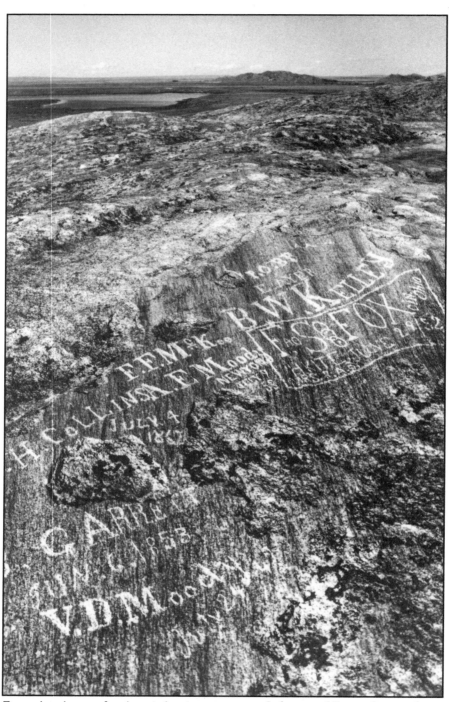

Expansive views and emigrant signatures are rewards for scrambling to the top of Independence Rock. Photo courtesy of the Wyoming Division of Tourism.

a scenic byway through the Seminoe Mountains, the jagged peaks that rise up southwest of Casper. The northern access is at Alcova, and the scenic byway is described in detail in the Back Country Byways guide from Falcon Press.

Check the gas gauge at Alcova before continuing west on Highway 220. It's forty-three miles to the next filling station at Muddy Gap Junction.

INDEPENDENCE ROCK

One of the most famous sights along the Oregon Trail, **Independence Rock**, is located fifty miles southwest of Casper, rising like a turtle or whale above the desert. During pioneer days, Independence Rock was as a landmark, lookout, campsite, trail register, and bulletin board. Today, it serves as backdrop for a conveniently located Wyoming state rest area and interpretive site along Highway 220.

To fully appreciate Independence Rock, however, visitors should climb to the top. It only takes about twenty minutes up and back, although most will want to spend more time enjoying the expansive views and emigrant signatures. In 1860, Sir Richard Burton calculated that 40,000 to 50,000 autographs had been placed on the rock in the previous decades. Most either chiseled their names or wrote them with a mixture of pine tar, gunpowder, and hog fat. Although most signatures have worn away, some are still visible, both at the top and within sheltered areas elsewhere on the rock, particularly on the south side. While on top, look for the Sweetwater River—which would guide the emigrants to South Pass—and for Devil's Gate, both to the west.

Howard Stansbury, who passed by on July 31, 1949, noted the rock "was covered with the names of passing emigrants, some of whom seemed determined, judging from the size of their inscriptions, that they would go down in posterity in all their fair proportions." Some trail entrepreneurs made money chiseling or writing autographs for their illiterate companions, charging up to five dollars depending on the signature's location.

John Fremont, seeing all the names in 1842, thought the rock was actually a large gravestone. According to the government Writers Project of 1939, Fremont decided to honor the dead by placing a large cross on the rock. Later, some migrants hostile to Roman Catholicism dynamited the section where Fremont had left the cross, which they looked upon as a symbol of the Catholic "sect."

Most stories on the naming of Independence Rock credit the fur trappers who traveled through the area before the Oregon-bound emigrants. One tale holds that a group of traders celebrated the Fourth of July at the rock in 1824. Another version maintains that William Sublette, leader of the first wagon train to the Continental Divide, spent July 4, 1830, at the

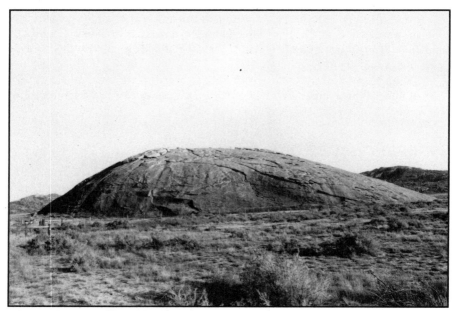

Many emigrants celebrated at Independence Rock because they were almost halfway to Oregon. Julie Fanselow photo.

rock and so named it in honor of the nation's birthday. However it was named, travelers by the time of the Oregon emigration looked forward to Independence Rock as a place to celebrate, whether or not they arrived on the Fourth of July. By now, they'd moved 814 miles from Independence, Missouri. They were almost halfway to Oregon.

Many emigrants mentioned Independence Rock in their journals. Robert Canfield visited on the Fourth of July, 1847, and noted that his party fired a cannon from atop the rock and planted a flag there. E.W. Conyers, describing a Fourth of July celebration in 1852, had this to say: "No person left the table hungry. After our feast, patriotic songs were indulged in, winding up with three cheers for Uncle Sam and three for Old Glory...a Fourth of July on the plains never to be forgotten."

A few miles past Independence Rock, the travelers marveled at **Devil's Gate**, a nasty-looking chasm carved through solid granite by the Sweetwater River. Wagons couldn't go through the gap and passed to the south, but some emigrants hiked over to view it up close. According to Arapahoe-Shoshone legend, a powerful evil spirit in the form of a big beast with tusks once wandered the Sweetwater Valley, preventing Indians from hunting or camping. A prophet told the tribes that the Great Spirit wanted them to destroy the beast, so they launched an attack from

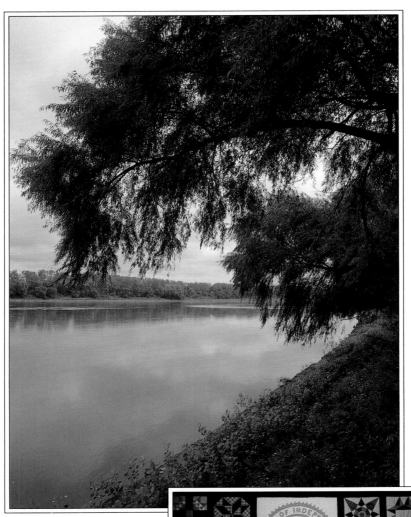

The Missouri River meanders past La Benite Park, Missouri, about three miles upstream from Independence Landing where emigrants began their trek west along the Oregon Trail. Photo by Gary Ladd.

A visitor admires one of the displays inside the National Frontier Trails Center in Independence, Missouri. Photo courtesy of the Missouri Division of Tourism.

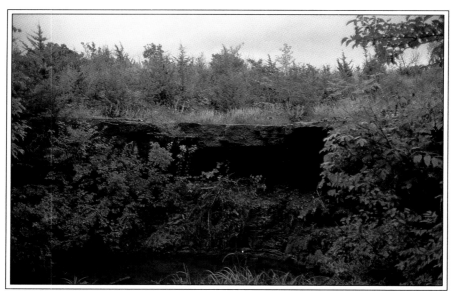

Alcove Springs near Marysville, Kansas, was a favorite rest stop along the trail. Photo by Julie Fanselow.

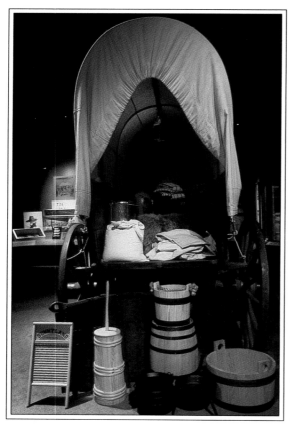

On display at the Kansas Museum of History in Topeka is a covered wagon full of supplies that visitors can unpack and repack, simulating the daily routine of families on the Oregon Trail. Photo courtesy of the Topeka Convention and Visitors Bureau.

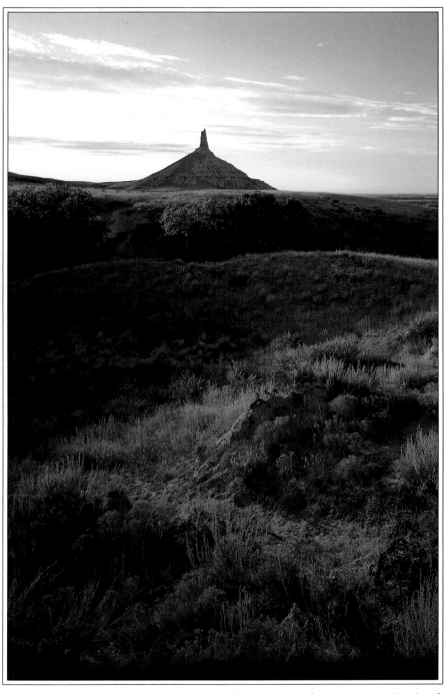

Chimney Rock, Nebraska, is now a national historic site and was once a navigational landmark along the trail. Photo by Gary Ladd.

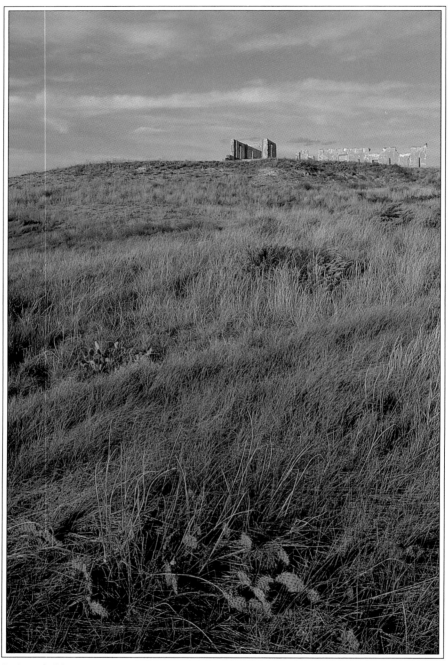

Ruins of old Fort Laramie, Wyoming, (not to be confused with the town of the same name) sit atop a hill. The fort was an important military post on the Oregon Trail. Photo by Joe Bensen.

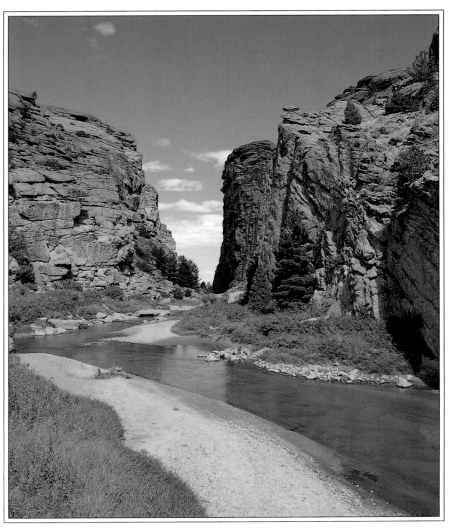

The Sweetwater River slices through a ridge of granite at Devil's Gate, Wyoming, near the Oregon Trail. Photo by Gary Ladd.

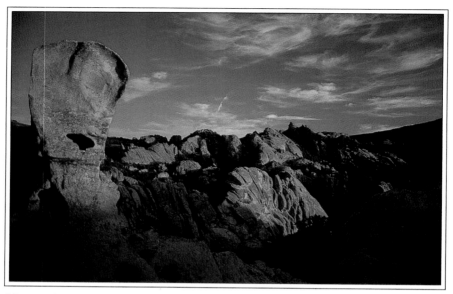

Many emigrants on their
way to the California gold
fields began their westward
trek on the Oregon Trail and
took a branch trail through
the City of Rocks to connect
up with the California Trail.
Photo by Randall Green.

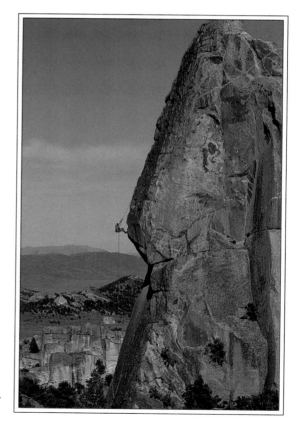

Today, the City of Rocks is a
popular destination for rock
climbers, hikers and sightseers.
Photo by Randall Green.

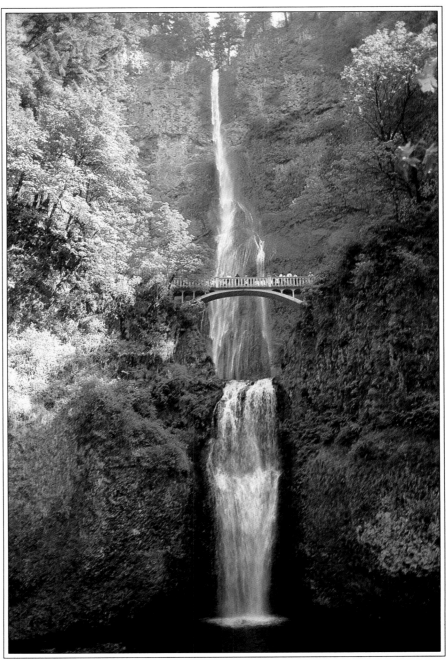

Multnomah Falls cascades into the Columbia River near the trail.
Photo by Julie Fanselow.

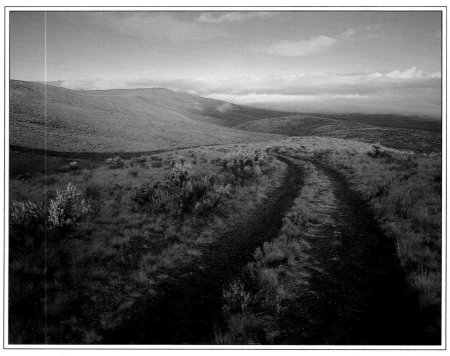

Old wagon ruts of the Oregon Trail descend a hill toward Virtue Flat near Baker City, Oregon. Photo by Gary Ladd.

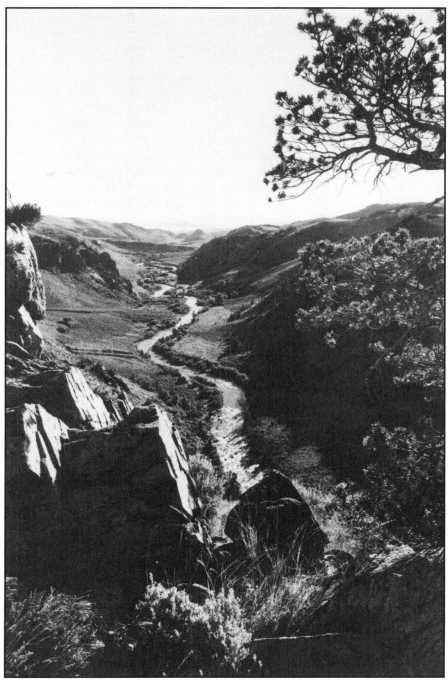
This view of the Sweetwater River gives one a sense of how the terrain became more rugged the farther west the emigrants traveled.
Photo courtesy of the Wyoming Division of Tourism.

nearby mountain passes and ravines, shooting countless arrows into the animal. The enraged creature, with a mighty upward thrust of its tusks, ripped a gap in the mountains, disappeared through the opening, and was never seen again.

Devil's Gate is now on private property, but the BLM has established an interpretive area six miles from Independence Rock offering a pretty good view, especially through binoculars or a telephoto lens. The BLM site also provides a glimpse of the Sun Ranch, one of Wyoming's largest. Visitors are alerted to the presence of Indian and emigrant graves nearby, and a monument tells about the tragedy of the Martin's Cove two miles northwest, where an exhausted group of Mormon handcart emigrants sought shelter from an early winter storm in 1856. Of 576 people in the company, 145 died before rescue parties from Salt Lake City could reach them.

Another turnout area west of Devil's Gate offers opportunities to see pronghorn, the antelope-like animals that can run up to seventy miles per hour. According to a display at the site, the pronghorn population once dwindled down to 5,000 animals. But the state prohibited hunting of the species between 1908 and 1915, and the pronghorn rapidly recovered. Today, there are about a half-million pronghorn, and two-thirds of the world's pronghorn population lives within a 300 mile radius of Casper.

Muddy Gap Junction marks the end of Highway 220. From here, U.S. Route 287 leads south to Rawlins and north to Lander (and on to Yellowstone and Grand Teton national parks). Turn right and head north.

Eleven-and-a-half miles from the junction, the BLM has another interpretive site, this one telling about **Split Rock**, the notch landmark that has been visible since Devil's Gate. Another turnout two miles west offers another view of the split and of the "Old Castle" or "Castle Rock," a smaller landmark south of the trail and highway.

The **Ice Spring Slough**, located 9.5 miles west of Jeffrey City, amazed and delighted the emigrants. Here, travelers could dig down a couple feet and discover ice, even in the searing summer heat. Peat-like turf once covered this marsh, insulating the frozen water beneath the surface. Today, the slough is nearly dry and little ice forms in the winter, but the area is still moist enough to produce occasional beautiful displays of wildflowers. The site is marked by a turnout and sign.

Jeffrey City, a once-booming uranium town that is now only slightly bigger than Muddy Gap Junction, offers another oasis on beautiful but remote Highway 287. Be cautious when driving this route in late summer—the setting sun glares against the windshield, and deer and pronghorn play on the roadside. Sweetwater Station, a rest area at the intersection of routes 287 and 135, has an excellent Oregon Trail map and display from the Fremont County Historical Society.

From here, the trail is about two miles south, paralleling the high-way. Most travelers will want to continue northwest to the intersection with Wyoming Highway 28, the route to South Pass. But those with time and inclination can drive the Hudson-Atlantic City Road, which follows the trail more closely. The maintained dirt road is open June through October. It turns south from Highway 287 about six miles west of Sweetwater Station and leads to the South Pass-Atlantic City historic mining district (which also is accessible via Highway 28). For more information about trail access or road conditions, contact the BLM's Lander office at (307) 332-7822.

Lander makes a fine spot to spend the night before continuing on to South Pass and Fort Bridger. A town of about 8,000 people, Lander lives for the outdoors. It's a major gateway to Grand Teton and Yellowstone national parks, the Wind River Range, and vast tracts of national forest. Sinks Canyon State Park, located nine miles southwest of town, features the beautiful Popo Agie River (pronounced Po-PO-zsha), a couple of great nature trails, and one of the most pleasant state park campgrounds you'll find anywhere. The park was named for the way the Popo Agie suddenly disappears into a large cavern before reappearing about a half-mile down the river canyon.

The Wind River Indian Reservation, home to the Shoshone and Arapahoe tribes, is north of Lander. Special events on the reservation include a Labor Day pow wow at Fort Washakie, rodeos throughout the summer, and three days of sun dances in July. Sacajawea, the Shoshone woman who guided Lewis and Clark, is buried on the reservation, as is Chief Washakie, a Shoshone chief who was the first Indian ever buried with military honors.

Lander also is home to the National Outdoor Leadership School, which teaches people how to tread lightly on the land. Visit the Lander Chamber of Commerce at 160 N. First St., or call (307) 332-3892 for more information on activities and sights in the area.

SIDETRIP: YELLOWSTONE AND GRAND TETON NATIONAL PARKS

Wyoming is blessed with Grand Teton and Yellowstone national parks, two of America's most spectacular natural areas. Grand Teton is a 132-mile drive northwest of Lander, and Yellowstone is another sixty miles north. A detour through these parks may well be in order, or better yet, plan another vacation to savor the magic that is northwest Wyoming.

Few people forget their first sight of the Tetons, which are among the youngest mountains in North America. These soaring, craggy peaks provide the setting for some of the greatest hiking in the world. The Cascade Canyon Trail is among the most popular treks, and the hikes to Hermitage Point or on the Paintbrush Trail often rewards visitors with wildlife views. Mountain climbing instruction and guides are available.

It's difficult to pull one's gaze away from the mountains, but the lakes and Snake River are lovely too. Activities include scenic boat trips, boat rentals, sailboarding on Jackson Lake, and floats down the Snake. Horseback riding, fishing, and camping offer still more pleasures.

Yellowstone was the world's first national park, so declared by President U.S. Grant in 1872. Known for its geysers, waterfalls, and wildlife (not to mention the 1988 fires that burned more than a third of the park), Yellowstone is among the most frequently visited national parks, so it can be crowded. Still, Yellowstone is a big place, with more than a thousand miles of trails. Solitude is available for those who seek it out. Yellowstone is mostly in Wyoming, although Idaho and Montana share narrow strips of the park's northwest corner.

Yellowstone boasts so many spectacular sights that it's hard to know where to begin. Artist Point and Inspiration Point offer vistas of the Grand Canyon of the Yellowstone River and its famous falls. Old Faithful is but one example of the park's intense thermal activity, all triggered by an immense volcanic eruption 600,000 years ago. Norris Geyser Basin and the Fountain Paint Pots area offer the park's most concentrated displays of these steaming, bubbling natural features.

Sightseeing is definitely the main attraction at Yellowstone. But other opportunities available include fishing (it's free, but a permit is required), backcountry camping and hiking, and canoeing (especially on Shoshone Lake). Power boaters are permitted on Yellowstone and Lewis lakes. One $10 vehicle permit is good for entrance at both Grand Teton and Yellowstone national parks. Senior citizens 62 and older and permanently disabled people are eligible for free passports good at these and all other national parks.

The town of Jackson sits south of Grand Teton National Park. Like other mountain resort towns, Jackson has gone through a lot of changes in recent decades. It no longer qualifies as a "typical" Western town, but it certainly is a fun place to visit. Jackson crackles with energy, from its creative restaurants and lively nightlife (don't miss the famous Million Dollar Cowboy Bar) to its wide recreational menu and active arts scene.

Another northwest Wyoming town, Cody, is famous for the Buffalo Bill Historical Center, considered by many to be the best overall Western museum in the United States. The four-part complex includes the Buffalo Bill Museum, which documents Col. William Cody's colorful life; the Whitney Gallery of Western Art, featuring original works by such famous names as Russell and Remington; the Plains Indian Museum, with extensive displays on the life and times of the region's great tribes; and the Winchester Gun Museum, which actually includes firearms from throughout history. Cody is eighty miles east of the Fishing Bridge junction at Yellowstone National Park.

For more information, contact Grand Teton National Park at (307) 733-2880; Yellowstone National Park at (307) 344-7381; the Jackson Hole Area Chamber of Commerce at (307) 733-3316; or the Cody Country Chamber at (307) 587-2297.

SOUTH PASS

As mountain passes go, **South Pass** wasn't much to look at in the nineteenth century, and it still isn't today. Many emigrants figured they'd be crossing through "a narrow defile in the Rocky Mountains walled in by perpendicular rocks hundreds of feet high," as Lorenzo Sawyer wrote in 1850. "The fact is they are in the South Pass all the way up the Sweetwater."

Because South Pass hardly looks like a mountain pass, emigrants who crossed the Continental Divide here scarcely knew they'd done so until they saw water flowing the "wrong" way on the other side. But the broad rise, twenty-nine miles wide, was the key to the whole Oregon Trail. It was the only place that allowed an easy passage through the Rocky Mountains, thus enabling wagons to roll over the divide with a minimum of difficulty. Aside from that, South Pass marked the emigrants' arrival in what was then Oregon Territory. Although travelers were only halfway to their destination, the pass was an important psychological benchmark.

South Pass was known and used by Indians for a long time before white men came along. Robert Stuart led his Astorian party through the area in 1812 as the party returned from the Pacific coast. A party of mountain men including Jim Bridger and Jed Smith rediscovered the way in 1824. A wagon train led by Capt. Benjamin Bonneville rolled through in 1832. Just over a decade later, the great emigration was on, with about 1,000 people traversing the pass in 1843.

Emigrants rarely stopped at the pass, although many made note of it in their journals. Kit Carson guided John Fremont's party through in 1842, and Fremont wrote: "The ascent had been so gradual that, with all the intimate knowledge possessed by Carson, who had made this country his home for seventeen years, we were obliged to watch very closely to find the place at which we had reached the culminating point."

Some writers grasped the full impact of the crossing. One emigrant woman, writing poetically of her party's last crossing of the Sweetwater River, noted they "forever took leave of the waters running toward the home of our childhood and youth." Another diarist, Theodore Talbot, said only: "Today we set foot in Oregon Territory...'The land of promise' as yet only promises an increased supply of wormwood and sand."

Although it is barely interpreted, South Pass is definitely worth a visit. And while an exhibit along Wyoming Highway 28 provides a good

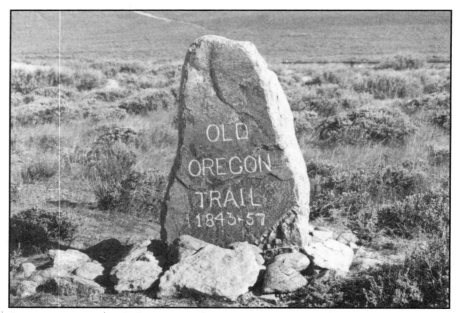

Stone monuments mark the summit of South Pass. Julie Fanselow photo.

view of the pass, it is easy enough to drive to the real thing and see it up close. The access road is forty-two miles south of Lander and ten miles south of the Willow Creek Inn. (A turnoff twenty-six miles south of Lander is the start of a loop road leading to Atlantic City and South Pass City, two old mining towns worth a visit while en route to South Pass itself. See descriptions below. This loop road leads back to Highway 28 near the Willow Creek Inn.)

Just before the turnoff, the highway crosses the Sweetwater River a final time and climbs. At the crest, .7 mile past the bridge, watch for a sign for the Bridger Wilderness (on the right when heading south). Turn left instead, onto Oregon Buttes Road. Drive about 2.75 miles to an old railroad bed. Drive another .4 mile to a "Y," bear right, then immediately right again. In another .2 mile, bear right yet again. South Pass is just ahead, past the cattle guard .6 mile away. Park by the cattle guard and stroll into history.

The pass is marked only by two small monuments. The one reading "Old Oregon Trail 1843-57" was placed on the continental divide by Ezra Meeker, the pioneer who went west in 1852 and later returned to mark the route. The other stone honors Narcissa Whitman and Eliza Spalding, first white women to cross the pass.

Near the pass, take time to look at the landscape, which has changed little since pioneer times. Here, the travelers had a natural corridor to follow, flanked on the north by the Wind River Range, its towering peaks cloaked in snow even in summer, and to the south by the Oregon Buttes and Antelope Hills.

From the pass, return to Highway 28. The roadside exhibit five miles south offers another perspective on the South Pass area. It also points out **Pacific Springs**, where the emigrants often camped after crossing the divide. The springs are now on private land.

Another five miles down Highway 28, a group of historical markers tell about the **"Parting of the Ways,"** the first of many major divisions in the trail where emigrants branched off to their various destinations. The actual jumping-off onto the Sublette Cutoff was eight miles west of this site; another turnout eight miles northwest of Farson on U.S. Highway 191 marks the route as it entered the Little Colorado Desert.

The Sublette Cutoff was opened in 1844 by a California-bound wagon train, but it didn't become popular until the gold rush of 1849. It originally was known as the Greenwood Cutoff (for one of the pioneering wagon train's guides, 81-year-old Caleb Greenwood), but an 1849 guidebook error forever changed its name. Although the Sublette Cutoff saved the travelers eighty-five miles and five or six days of travel, it was tough going, with dry stretches and mountainous terrain.

Farson, at the junction of Highway 28 and U.S. 191, is a good pit stop for today's traveler. Gas, food, and lodging are available, not to mention what may be the biggest ice cream cones in Wyoming at the Farson Merc. Present-day Farson also is where the main Oregon Trail crossed the Big Sandy River before following its north bank to the Green River. Here, Jim Bridger and Brigham Young met for the first time in 1847. Bridger gave Young a description of the Salt Lake Valley, which the mountain man was credited with discovering in 1824. In return, Young gave Bridger a free pass for the the Platte River ferry at Casper. A plaque by the Big Sandy bridge commemorates the encounter.

From Farson, stay close to the trail by driving Highway 28 to Wyoming Highway 372, then take Highway 372 south to I-80. This route passes near the Seedskadee National Wildlife Refuge, famous for its wide variety of birds.

Alternatively, travel south on U.S. Highway 191 to I-80 and the Rock Springs-Green River area, the biggest metropolitan region in western Wyoming with a population of about 35,000. Rock Springs started out in 1862 as a stop on the Overland Stage route, and it remains an important transportation center. To the north, the Red Desert region stretches more than 100 miles and serves as home to one of the nation's largest wild horse populations. The Bureau of Land Management controls the herd's size by rounding up some of the animals and offering them for adoption.

Visitors aren't allowed to watch the wild horse roundups, but they are welcome at the Red Desert Roundup, a major rodeo held each July. Arts-minded travelers may want to stop at the Rock Springs Community

Fine Arts Center, located in the public library at 400 "C" St. This collection includes hundreds of works by Wyoming and other Western artists. The local Recreation Center at Reagan Avenue and Sweetwater Drive has year-round sports facilities open to the public.

Rock Springs and Green River are known for their nearby deposits of trona, used to make soda ash, which in turn is used to produce glass, detergents, and baking soda. Two-thirds of the world's soda ash comes from southwest Wyoming. Green River is the seat of Sweetwater County and home of the local historical museum at 80 W. Flaming Gorge Way. Its exhibits include a large collection of historical photographs from the region.

Both towns abound in visitor services and serve as gateways to Flaming Gorge National Recreation Area. For more information, contact the Rock Springs Chamber of Commerce at (307) 362-3771 or the Green River Chamber of Commerce at (307) 875-5711. From Green River, it's about an hour's drive west on I-80 to Fort Bridger.

SIDETRIP: SOUTH PASS CITY AND ATLANTIC CITY

After Oregon Trail travel tapered off with the coming of the transcontinental railroad, the South Pass region was the scene of much mining activity. South Pass City was built north of the Oregon Trail in 1867 after the Carissa Mine struck a rich vein of gold. The town's population boomed to 2,000 people within a year, and more than thirty mines started working the hillsides. The bust hit in 1872, and most folks moved away.

South Pass City is now a state historic park with twenty-four structures still intact (out of about 300 that once existed). Summer activities include living history displays and one of Wyoming's oldest and largest Fourth of July celebrations. Visitors can buy gold-panning equipment and try their luck in nearby Willow Creek, tour the remaining buildings, or enjoy a picnic lunch on the pleasant grounds. Buildings are open from 9 a.m. to 6 p.m. daily May 15 through Oct. 15, and the grounds are open year-round. For more information, call (307) 332-3684.

A museum in the visitor center tells the town's history, including its substantial role in the women's rights movement: In 1869, South Pass City's representative in the Wyoming territorial legislature, William Bright, introduced a bill giving women the rights to vote, to run for office, and to hold property. It passed, making Wyoming was the first state or territory to extend these rights to women and leading to its nickname, "the Equality State." Two months later, Esther Morris was appointed South Pass City's first justice of the peace and the nation's first female judge.

South Pass City isn't quite a ghost town. A baby was born to a resident as recently as 1990, and toys strewn about one pleasant yard attest to the fact a few families still live here. (The 1992 population was set at fifteen.) South Pass is also home to Trails West, a wagon trail outfitting company run by Bill and Nona Bates. Their popular three-day covered wagon treks run June through August, leaving Tuesday morning and returning Thursday evening. En route, participants see many pioneer sites and experience what life was like on the trail. One-day horseback trips, wildlife photo pack trips, and chuck wagon dinners are offered, too. For more information, write Trails West at 65 Main Street, South Pass City, WY 82520, or call (800) 327-4052.

Atlantic City, another old gold camp, is just northeast of South Pass City. The town was so named because it was located east of the Continental Divide. It too has escaped becoming a complete ghost town, with several small businesses catering to the tourist trade. The Atlantic City Mercantile features live music on summer weekends, as well as food. The whole family is welcome. The Miner's Delight Inn is a bed-and-breakfast widely known for its fine dining. (Reservations are necessary for either meals or lodging; phone (307) 332-3513.) Campers will find two BLM campgrounds near Atlantic City, and a few cabins are available in town, too. Make sure to have a jacket or sweater handy when visiting South Pass City or Atlantic City. Elevations are near 8,000 feet, and the area gets some of Wyoming's harshest weather year-round.

The Shoshone National Forest west of Highway 28 is another favorite recreational area, particularly for Wyomingites who want to avoid the crowds that often congregate at their state's national parks. Fiddler's Lake and Louis Lake are among the popular spots in this scenic area. For information, call the forest headquarters at (307) 527-6921 or stop by the turnout on the west side of the highway about thirty miles south of Lander.

FORT BRIDGER

By the early 1840s, the fur-trading days of the American West were coming to a close, and Jim Bridger needed something new to occupy his time. He decided to build a fort to capitalize on the coming westward migration, a place where emigrants could buy supplies, fix their wagons, and rest before resuming their trips. His first post was situated almost a mile north of the present-day town of Fort Bridger; a second fort, erected in 1844, was on the ground now occupied by **Fort Bridger State Historic Site.**

By most accounts, Fort Bridger wasn't a pretty place. In *The Oregon Trail Revisited,* Gregory Franzwa described the post as "a raunchy adobe emplacement surrounded by a stockade—always a disappointment to trail-weary emigrants." But, as Franzwa noted, what the fort lacked in aesthetic appeal it made up for by its surroundings. Emigrant diarists wrote of abundant clear, sweet water and good grass for their livestock.

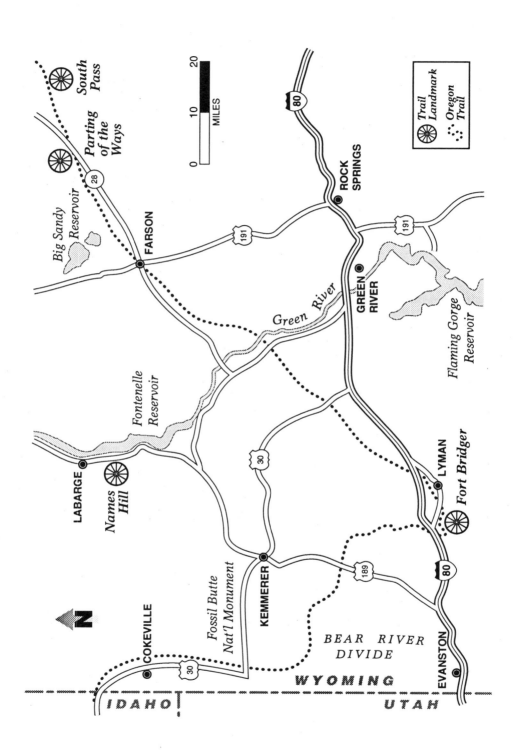

They also couldn't help but notice the beautiful Uinta Mountains to the south, nor the high, wide blue skies that prevailed then and now over Wyoming.

Despite their new roles as shopkeepers, Bridger and Vasquez were still mountain men at heart, and some visitors to the fort reported the proprietors were nowhere to be found. When they did stick around, however, Bridger and Vasquez received good notices from their patrons. James Reed, who stopped by in July 1846, called them "two very excellent and accommodating gentlemen...they can be relied on for doing business honorably and fairly."

Some other deals that went down here were shadier; Fort Bridger was to be the rendezvous site for Lansford Hastings and the Donner party, which he had promised to lead on his new shortcut to California. When George Donner and his party arrived, Hastings had already moved on. The party used the Hastings route anyway, following his tracks. Within days, however, the Donner party had lost the way. Three months later, they found themselves trapped by an early blizzard in the Sierra Mountains of California.

Fort Bridger also played a pivotal role for members of the Church of Jesus Christ of Latter-day Saints, or Mormons, who were headed for religious freedom in what would become Utah. This, in fact, was the point where the Mormon Trail—which had paralleled the Oregon Trail since Fort Kearny—left the track bound for Oregon and California and struck off southwest toward the Great Salt Lake. About 70,000 Mormons followed the trail from Nauvoo, Illinois, to Salt Lake City between 1847 and 1869, many of them using handcarts instead of covered wagons. From their base in Salt Lake City, the Mormons went on to settle more than 300 communities in the West.

The Mormons ended up buying Fort Bridger in 1855, but the occupation was destined to be short-lived, lasting only two years. Tensions mounted between the Mormons and the federal government, and President Buchanan sent troops to the area in 1857. Rather than fight, the Mormons burned Fort Bridger and their nearby Fort Supply and retreated to Salt Lake City.

From 1858 on, Fort Bridger became a military site and remained so until its final abandonment in 1890. Soldiers rebuilt the fort, and it is these Army-era buildings that are the site's main attractions today. Visitors can easily walk the grounds and tour several buildings and the fort museum in about an hour. The museum features good displays on all aspects of the fort's history, from the Oregon Trail to the military to its use by Indians.

One of the most fascinating characters in Fort Bridger history was William A. Carter, who started as a sutler at the trading post and went on to become a judge, living here until his death in 1881. Carter's clan enjoyed comforts known by few other frontier families, including one of the region's largest libraries. Today's Fort Bridger is especially well

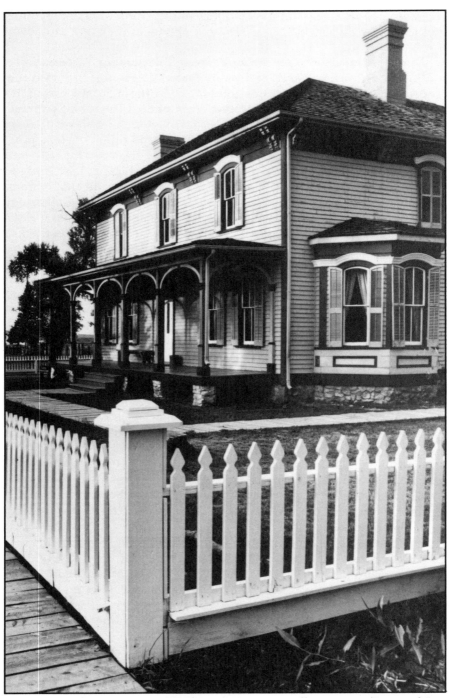

The officers' quarters at Fort Bridger State Historic Site offer a unique glimpse of the past. Photo courtesy of the Wyoming Division of Tourism.

suited for handicapped people, with its flat walkways and Braille signs provided by the Lions Club from the nearby town of Lyman.

Modern-day Fort Bridger also includes a replica of the Bridger-Vasquez trading post. Tucked back in the site's northwest corner, the post stocks fur-trade and emigrant-era goods such as skins, pelts, beads, and hats. The shop is run by Dick and Sandy Gregory, a couple who live in the adjacent cabin and spend their off-season traveling to different mountain-man and fur-trader rendezvous. Fort Bridger itself hosts one of the nation's biggest such gatherings each Labor Day Weekend. The rendezvous, with associated events including a demolition derby and other entertainment, attracts thousands of participants and onlookers.

Fort Bridger State Historic Site is open all year and is located near Exit 34 off I-80. The museum is open from 8:30 a.m. to 5:30 p.m. daily June through Labor Day and from 9 a.m. to 4:30 p.m. Saturdays and Sundays during the rest of the year. The Bridger-Vasquez Trading Post is open May through September. For more information, call (307) 782-3842.

Visitor services are available in the town of Fort Bridger and nearby communities including Lyman and Mountain View. From Fort Bridger, the Oregon Trail turned north toward present-day Idaho. Modern travelers can backtrack on I-80 to Wyoming Highway 412, follow it north to its junction with U.S. Highway 189, then drive north to Kemmerer, home of the first J.C. Penney store and a fine little museum (the Fossil Country Frontier Museum at 400 Pine Avenue). Evanston, twenty-eight miles west of Fort Bridger, is another possible overnight stop; from Evanston, backtrack thirteen miles east to U.S. Highway 189 and drive north to Kemmerer. From Kemmerer, take U.S. Highway 30 fifty-five miles west then north into Idaho.

SIDETRIP: FLAMING GORGE, FOSSIL BUTTE, AND DINOSAUR COUNTRY

A detour off Interstate 80 leads to Flaming Gorge National Monument, a spectacular area of bright red canyons, towering green ponderosa pines, and abundant recreational opportunities. The most scenic route through the area is U.S. Highway 191, which heads south between Rock Springs and Green River.

Fishing and boating are the most popular activities at Flaming Gorge, which was named by Major John Wesley Powell during his explorations of the area in 1869. Numerous boat and tackle rental shops dot the area near the Wyoming-Utah border. The Flaming Gorge Dam Visitor Center at Dutch John offers tours, self-guiding maps, and coloring books for the kids. The Red Canyon Visitor Center on Utah Highway 44 boasts a spectacular quarter-mile-high vista above the lake and canyon. Primitive camping is available here too. For more information, call (801) 889-3713.

Dinosaur fans young and old will enjoy a side trip to Dinosaur National Monument, about 12 miles south of I-80 at Jensen, Utah. (Take Utah Highway 149 from Jensen to the site.) Fossilized bones from brontosaurus and other prehistoric creatures were found here in one of the largest concentrations anywhere in the world. A visitor center displays many bones and related exhibits. Admission to the monument is $5 per vehicle. Call (801) 789-2115 for more information.

Prehistoric life is also the focus at Fossil Butte National Monument, ten miles west of Kemmerer, Wyoming. During the Eocene Age 50 million years ago, this area was covered with a freshwater lake. As the lake dried up, it left behind a wealth of beautifully fossilized fish and other aquatic creatures. The area is a geological wonderland, with its buff-colored Green River Formation layers mingling with the red, pink, and purple Wasatch Formation.

The monument's new visitor center exhibits a variety of fossils and an artist's rendition of what the area might have looked like during prehistoric times. A 2.5-mile trail leads to the area where the fossils were quarried. The visitor center is open daily from 8 a.m. to 7 p.m. June through August and from 8 a.m. to 4:30 p.m. the rest of the year. Grounds are open year-round. Admission to the monument is free. For more information, call (307) 877-4455.

LODGING

TORRINGTON, WYOMING

Maverick Motel, (307) 532-4064, Routes 26 and 85, $29.

Oregon Trail Lodge, (307) 532-2101, 710 E. Valley Road.

Western Motel, (307) 532-2104, U.S. Highway 26, $34.

GUERNSEY, WYOMING

Annette's White House Bed & Breakfast, (307) 836-2148, 239 South Dakota St.

Bunkhouse Hotel, (307) 836-2356, U.S. Highway 26.

Sage Brush Motel, (307) 836-2331.

GLENDO, WYOMING

Bellwood Motel, (307) 735-4211, Yellowstone Highway.

Howard's Motel, (307) 735-4252, 106 ""A" St.

DOUGLAS, WYOMING

Akers Ranch Bed & Breakfast, (307) 358-3741, 81 Inez Road.

Chieftain Motel, (307) 358-2673, 815 E. Richards St., $29.

Holiday Inn, (800) HOLIDAY, 1450 Riverbend Drive, $61.

Super 8 Motel, (800) 843-1991, 314 Russell Ave., $34.

Winchester Inn, (307) 358-4780, 2310 E. Richards St.

GLENROCK, WYOMING

All-American Inn, (307) 436-2772, 500 W. Aspen, $19-$29.

Coachman Motel, (307) 436-2281, 108 S. 3rd St.

Hotel Higgins, (307) 436-9212, 416 W. Birch St., $52.

CASPER, WYOMING

Best Western East, (800) 528-1234, 2325 E. Yellowstone Highway, $43-$58.

Casper Hilton Inn, (800) HILTONS, 800 N. Poplar, $64-$78.

Durbin Street Inn Bed & Breakfast, (307) 577-5774, 843 S. Durbin St.

I-25 Inn, (307)234-9125, I-25 and Wyoming Blvd., $30.

La Quinta Motor Inn, (307) 234-1159, 301 E. ""E" St., $45-$51.

Sage and Sand Motel, (307) 237-2088, 901 W. Yellowstone Highway.

Showboat Motel, (307) 235-2711, $31.

Travelier Motel, (307) 237-9343, 500 E. First, $20.

Westridge Motel, 307) 234-8911, 955 CY Ave., $28-$32.

BESSEMER BEND AREA, WYOMING

Bessemer Bend Bed & Breakfast, (307) 265-6819, ten miles west of Casper at 5120 Alcova Road.

LANDER, WYOMING

Budget Host Pronghorn Lodge, (307) 332-3940, 150 E. Main St., $40.

Country Fare Bed & Breakfast, (307) 332-5906, 904 Main St.

Downtown Motel, (307) 332-5220, 569 Main St.

Maverick Motel, (307) 332-2821, 808 Main St.

Silver Spur Motel, (307) 332-5189, 340 N. 10th, $32.

Teton Motel, (307) 332-3582, 586 Main St.

ATLANTIC CITY, WYOMING

Miner's Delight Inn, (307) 332-3513.

FARSON, WYOMING

Sitzman's Motel, (307) 273-9241.

ROCK SPRINGS, WYOMING

American Family Inn, (800) 548-6621, 1635 N. Elk St., $39.

Cody's Motel, (307) 362-6675, 75 N. Center St.

Holiday Inn, (800) HOLIDAY, 1675 Sunset Drive, $56-$63.

Inn at Rock Springs, (800) 442-9692, I-80 Exit 102, $55-$72.

Lamplighter Friendship Inn, (307) 362-6673, 1004 Dewar Drive, $30.

Motel 6, (307) 362-1850, 2615 Commercial Way.

Park Inn, (307) 362-9600, 2518 Foothill Blvd.

GREEN RIVER, WYOMING

Coachman Inn Motel, (307) 875-3681, 470 E. Flaming Gorge Way, $28-$30.

Desmond Motel, (307) 875-3701, 140 N. 7th, $28-$30.

GREEN RIVER, WYOMING (CONT.)

Super 8 Motel, (800) 843-1991, 208 W. Flaming Gorge Way, $37.

Western Motel, (307) 875-2840, 890 W. Flaming Gorge Way, $35-$37.

LITTLE AMERICA, WYOMING

Little America, (800) 634-2401, I-80 Exit 68, $48-$52.

LYMAN, WYOMING

Valley West Motel, (307) 787-3700, Main Street.

FORT BRIDGER, WYOMING

Wagon Wheel Motel, (307) 782-6361, located across from Fort Bridger State Historic Site.

EVANSTON, WYOMING

Classic Lodge, (307) 789-6830, 202 Highway 30 East, $30-$35.

Dunmar Inn, (800) 654-6509, 1601 Harrison Drive, $62-$74.

Pine Gables Lodge Bed & Breakfast, (307) 789-2069, 1049 Center St., $37.

Weston Lamplighter, (307) 789-0783, 1983 Harrison Drive, $50.

KEMMERER, WYOMING

Antler Motel, (307) 877-4461, 419 Coral St.

Burnett's New Motel, (307) 877-4471. 1326 Central Ave.

Energy Inn, Diamondville, (307) 877-6901.

Fairview Motel, (307) 877-3938, Routes 30 and 89, $44-$48.

Lazy U Motel, (307) 877-4428, 521 Coral St.

COKEVILLE, WYOMING

Valley Hi Motel, (307) 279-3251, Highway 30.

CAMPING

TORRINGTON, WYOMING

Kountry Kids, east of town on Highway 26.

Pioneer Municipal Park, W. 15th Ave. and ""E" St. Free.

Travelers Trailer Court & Campground, 750 Main St.

FORT LARAMIE, WYOMING

Bennett Court, (307) 837-2270, North Laramie Ave. at Highway 26.

Chuckwagon Drive-In Campground, (307) 837-2828, Fort Laramie.

Fort Laramie Municipal Park, (307) 837-2711, on Fort Laramie Avenue. Free.

K & K Kampground, between Lingle and Fort Laramie on Highway 26.

GUERNSEY, WYOMING

Guernsey State Park, (307) 836-2334, three miles north of Guernsey.

GLENDO, WYOMING

Collins Corral, south of town on Highway 319.

Glendo Marina, (307) 735-4216, 383 Glendo Park Road.

Glendo State Park, (307) 735-4433, four miles east of Glendo.

Lakeview Motel & Campground, (307) 735-4461, north edge of town.

DOUGLAS, WYOMING

Jackalope KOA, (307) 358-2164, I-25 Exit 140.

Several U.S. Forest Service campgrounds are located in the Medicine Bow National Forest south of Douglas. Call (307) 358-4690 for information.

AYRES NATURAL BRIDGE, WYOMING

Ayres Natural Bridge, I-25 Exit 146, then five miles south. Free.

CASPER, WYOMING

Beartrap Meadow/Casper Mountain, (307) 234-6821, seven miles south on Casper Mountain Road.

Casper KOA, (800) 423-5155, 2800 E. Yellowstone Highway. Kamping Kabins.

Casper Mountain Park, (307) 234-6821, six miles south on Casper Mountain Road.

Fort Caspar Campground, (307) 234-3260, west of Fort Caspar on 13th St.

P.M. Campgrounds, (307) 577-1664, 1101 Prairie Lane.

ALCOVA, WYOMING

Alcova Lake Campground, (307) 234-6821, thirty miles southwest of Casper on Highway 220.

Pathfinder Lake Campground, (307) 234-6821, seven miles south of Highway 220 on Pathfinder Road.

JEFFREY CITY, WYOMING

Cottonwood Campground, (307) 332-7822, six miles east on Highway 287, then eight miles south on Green Mountain BLM Road. Primitive sites.

LANDER, WYOMING

K-Bar Ranch, (307) 332-3836, ten miles southeast on Highway 287.

Ray Lake Campground, nine miles northwest on Highway 287.

Rocky Acres Camper and Trailer Park, (307) 332-6953, four miles northwest on Highway 287.

Sinks Canyon State Park, (307) 332-6333, six miles southwest on Highway 131.

Several Forest Service campgrounds are located in the Shoshone National Forest southwest of Lander. Check roadside display on Highway 28 or call (307) 332-5460 for information.

ATLANTIC CITY, WYOMING

Atlantic City BLM campgrounds, (307) 332-7822, twenty-eight miles south of Lander; follow signs from Highway 28. Primitive sites.

FARSON, WYOMING

Big Sandy State Recreation Area, (307) 332-3684, eight miles north on Highway 287, then two miles east on county road. Primitive sites.

ROCK SPRINGS, WYOMING

Albert's Trailer Court, 1560 Elk St. S.

Rock Springs KOA, (307) 362-3063, 86 Foothill Blvd. Kamping Kabins.

GREEN RIVER, WYOMING

Tex's Travel Camp, (307) 875-2630, between I-80 exits 85 and 89.

LYMAN, WYOMING

Lyman/Fort Bridger KOA, (307) 786-2762, I-80 Exit 413.

EVANSTON, WYOMING

Phillips RV & Trailer Park, (307) 789-3805, 225 Bear River Drive.

Sunset RV Park, (307) 789-3763, 196 Bear River Drive.

KEMMERER, WYOMING

Riverside Trailer Park, 216 Spinel St.

RESTAURANTS

TORRINGTON, WYOMING

Simar's Chinese & American Cuisine, (307) 532-8470, 1930 Main St.

LINGLE, WYOMING

Lira's Mexican Food, (307) 837-2826.

GUERNSEY, WYOMING

Crazy Tony's, (307) 836-2113, Highway 26.

GLENDO, WYOMING

Flying Dutchman Bar & Steakhouse, (307) 735-4279, 115 S. Yellowstone Ave.

DOUGLAS, WYOMING

Big Wheel Truck Stop, (307) 358-4446, east of Douglas off of I-25. Open 24 hours.

Chutes Wyoming Eatery, (307) 358-9790, in Holiday Inn, 1450 Riverbend Drive.

Country Inn, (307) 358-3575, 2341 E. Richards. Family dining.

GLENROCK, WYOMING

The Paisley Shawl, (307) 436-9212, in Hotel Higgins, 416 W. Birch St. Prime rib and steaks, Victorian atmosphere.

CASPER, WYOMING

Anthony's Italian Restaurant, (307) 234-3071, 241 S. Center St. Specializes in fresh pasta.

Benham's, (307) 234-4531, 739 N. Center. Varied menu features barbecue ribs.

Crazy Crab, (307) 266-3474, 144 S. Center. Daily fresh seafood.

CASPER, WYOMING (CONT.)

El Jarro Family Restaurant, (307) 577-0538, 500 W. "F" St. Homemade Mexican food.

Goose Egg Inn, (307) 473-8838, five miles southwest on Highway 220. Prime rib. Established in 1936.

J.B.'s Big Boy Restaurant, (307) 234-7301, 600 W. "F" St.

King's Table Buffet, (307) 577-6013, 111 Star Lane. Large buffet selection.

South Sea Chinese Restaurant, (307) 237-4777, 2025 E. 2nd St. Chinese and American cuisine.

ALCOVA, WYOMING

Alcova Lakeside Marina, (307) 472-6666, 24025 Lakeshore Drive. Restaurant, lounge, and grocery store.

JEFFREY CITY, WYOMING

Drillers Delight Restaurant & Lounge, (307) 544-2361.

LANDER, WYOMING

The Commons Restaurant, (307) 332-5149, 170 E. Main St. Steaks, prime rib, seafood.

The Hitching Rack, (307) 332-4322, Highway 287. Steaks and seafood.

Judd's Grub, (307) 332-9680, 634 Main. Drive-in style fast food.

Loft Restaurant, (307) 332-3102, Lander Mall. Thai-American cuisine.

ATLANTIC CITY, WYOMING

Atlantic City Mercantile, (307) 332-5143. Lunch daily; dinner Thursday-Saturday, specializing in "Aspen barbecue rib-eye steak."

Miner's Delight, (307) 332-3513. Breakfast and dinner Wednesday through Sunday. Reservations needed.

FARSON, WYOMING

Oregon Trail Cafe, (307) 273-9631. Local gathering spot.

ROCK SPRINGS, WYOMING

Key Largo Cafe, (307) 362-9600, in The Inn at Rock Springs. Sunday brunch.

Killpeppers, (307) 382-8012, 1030 Dewar Drive. Prime rib, steaks, seafood.

Mr. C's, (307) 382-9200, in the Holiday Inn, 1675 Sunset Drive. Continental cuisine.

Outlaw Inn Restaurant, (307) 362-6623, in the Best Western, 1630 Elk St. Western and gourmet dining.

Ted's Supper Club, (307) 362-7323, three miles west on I-80. Steak, seafood, chicken.

GREEN RIVER, WYOMING

Embers Family Restaurant, (307) 875-9983, 95 E. Railroad. Char-broiled steaks.

Red Feather Inn, (307) 875-6625, 211 E. Flaming Gorge. Lunch, dinner, lounge.

Rita's Fine Mexican Food, (307) 875-5503, 520 Willes Drive. Chile verde, other Mexican combo meals.

Trudel's Restaurant, (307) 875-8040, 3 E. Flaming Gorge Way.

LITTLE AMERICA, WYOMING

Little America Restaurant, I-80 Exit 68, (800) 634-2401. Open 24 hours.

LYMAN, WYOMING

Lyman Steak House and Drive-In, (307) 787-3110, 321 E. Clark St.

MOUNTAIN VIEW, WYOMING

Pizza Hut, (307) 782-6661, Highway 414.

URIE, WYOMING

Lotty's Family Restaurant, (307) 786-2287, Highway 414.

FORT BRIDGER, WYOMING

Pete & Patty's, (307) 782-9825, one block east of Fort Bridger State Historic Site.

Wagon Wheel Cafe, (307) 782-3585, located across from Fort Bridger State Historic Site.

EVANSTON, WYOMING

Dunmar's Legal Tender, (307) 789-3770, in the Best Western, 1601 Harrison Drive. Live entertainment.

Last Outpost, (307) 789-3322, 205 Bear River Drive. Ranch-raised buffalo steaks, chuck wagon fare.

Main Street Deli, (307) 789-1599, 1025 Main. Specialty sandwiches, soups, doughnuts.

KEMMERER, WYOMING

The Frontier Restaurant, (307) 877-9922, Highway 233.

Lake Viva Naughton Marina Restaurant, (307) 877-9669, fifteen miles north on Highway 233.

Luigi's, (307) 877-6221, 819 Susie Ave. (Diamondville). Steaks, seafood, Italian specialties.

Nishi's Corner Cafe, (307) 877-4007, 801 S. Main. Chinese and American food.

Polar King, (307) 877-9448, U.S. Highway 189. Breakfast anytime.

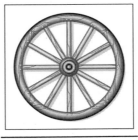

CHAPTER SIX

TOUGH GOING: IDAHO

"Traveled fifteen miles today over the most torturous road I ever could have imagined. Nothing but rock after rock ...nothing but sage."
—Emigrant Esther McMillan Hanna, 1852

SOUTHEAST IDAHO AND SODA SPRINGS

The pioneers had a curious saying to describe a key passage of their progress west. As parties started out, spirits were usually high. Eventually, however, the travelers would "see the elephant." This meant they had finally come face to face with the bitter realities of their journey—the untimely deaths, lost possessions, crazy weather, and tortuous terrain. And by the time they passed through Idaho, the emigrants had "seen the elephant" many times over.

Soon after entering present-day Idaho, the wagon trains had to ford the **Thomas Fork**, where steep, muddy inclines in and out of the stream made crossing most difficult. In 1850, emigrants built two bridges on the site, but a toll collector soon started charging for the bridges' use. The fee, a dollar per wagon, was more than many could afford by this point.

Just a few miles farther west, the emigrants came to a high ridge that became known as **"the Big Hill"** east of what is now Montpelier. Many pioneers thought this was the steepest, longest hill they'd yet seen. "The ascent is very long and tedious, but the descent is still more abrupt and

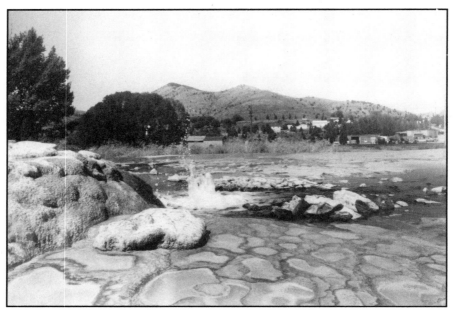

The geyser at Soda Springs is still an attraction to visitors. Julie Fanselow photo.

difficult," Theodore Talbot wrote in 1843. "It is about one mile to the plain, and generally very steep and stony, but all reached the plain safely and were truly thankful that they had safely passed one of the most difficult mountains on the road," Joel Palmer wrote in 1845. Many wagons were let down by ropes tied to trees that are now long gone. But the pioneers' hardships are still remembered at the Oregon Trail Rendezvous Pageant, re-enacted each year on the Friday closest to July 24. Area trail enthusiasts also hope to someday erect a National Oregon Trail Museum near the intersection of U.S. Highways 30 and 89 in Montpelier. The trail closely parallels U.S. 30 throughout this region.

Once in the Bear River Valley, travelers found a trading post established in 1848 by Thomas L. "Peg Leg" Smith, a mountain man from Utah who had to amputate his own leg twenty years before. In 1849, gold-seekers rushing to California passed here by the thousands, and Smith reportedly made $100 a day. No traces of the post remain.

But unquestionably, **Soda Springs** was the major attraction in the Bear River country. Here the emigrants marveled at springs, geysers, and a landscape marked by cones and craters formed by mineral deposits. "These soda springs are well worth a notice, possessing all the properties of pure soda water," emigrant Samuel Hancock wrote in 1845. William J. Scott, who passed through the area a year later, said he drank a whole

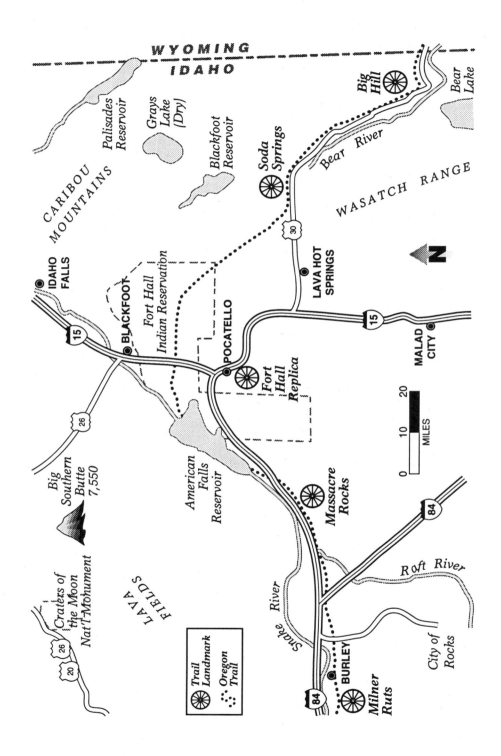

WYOMING

IDAHO

Palisades
Reservoir

Grays
Lake
(Dry)

Blackfoot
Reservoir

Soda
Springs

Bear River

Big
Hill

Bear
Lake

CARIBOU
MOUNTAINS

WASATCH RANGE

30

N

LAVA HOT
SPRINGS

IDAHO
FALLS

Fort Hall
Indian Reservation

15

15

MALAD
CITY

BLACKFOOT

POCATELLO

Fort
Hall
Replica

26

20

MILES

10

0

Big
Southern Butte
7,550

American Falls
Reservoir

Massacre
Rocks

84

Craters of
the Moon
Nat'l Monument

LAVA
FIELDS

Raft River

Snake River

City
of Rocks

26

Trail
Landmark

Oregon
Trail

20

BURLEY

Milner
Ruts

84

gallon of the stuff. The most popular site may have been the one known as Beer Spring. Rufus B. Sage, who visited in 1842, had this to say: "The draught will prove delicious and somewhat stimulating, but, if repeated too freely, it is said to produce a kind of giddiness like intoxication."

There once were more than 100 such springs in the area. Most have disappeared, but one, Hooper Spring, has been preserved at a city park north of the town of Soda Springs. To get there, turn right on Third Street East. Drive 1.5 miles north, then turn left and proceed to the park. The spring is located under a shady pavilion, and a plaque encourages visitors to "drink deeply of nature's best beverage." Visitors really can drink the water, which is full of such yummy ingredients as silica, iron, calcium, magnesium, and bicarbonate radicle.

Another spring regularly gave off a sound like that of a steamboat. It is now drowned beneath the reservoir, but it hasn't disappeared entirely. The best way to see it is to play nine holes at the Soda Springs Golf Club. Look south to the reservoir from either the No. 1 green or the No. 8 tee. On a calm day, watch for a slight disturbance on the water's surface. That is Steamboat Spring, still percolating and puffing away. The golf course also boasts a fine Oregon Trail swale that emerges from the lake, cuts across the No. 9 fairway, and skirts the No. 1 green before traversing the No. 8 fairway. This most unusual hazard, sometimes cursed by local golfers, has even made the pages of National Geographic.

The local cemetery was built around the Wagonbox Grave, which commemorates the deaths of eight members of an emigrant family who were allegedly killed by Indians in 1861. Nearby, the world's only captive geyser erupts for about five minutes every hour on the hour unless the wind is blowing in a westerly direction. The geyser, discovered in 1937 while officials were trying to find a hot-water source for the local swimming pool, is now capped and controlled by a timer. A small park across the street from the geyser offers a place to picnic or relax on the front-porch-style swings until the show begins.

West of Soda Springs, at a landmark called Sheep Rock or Soda Point, some emigrants left the main trail and struck west for California on a route that came to be known as Hudspeth's Cutoff. Originally used by Indians, the route became popular in 1849 even though it saved only two days' travel and twenty-five miles. The main trail set off on a northwesterly course before emerging north of present-day Pocatello at Fort Hall. No good roads parallel the trail through this mountainous region, but the modern route is absolutely delightful. Follow U.S. 30 east to Interstate 15. From the junction, it's just twenty miles to Pocatello and a fine Fort Hall replica.

SIDETRIP: BEAR LAKE AND LAVA HOT SPRINGS

Much of southern Idaho is a high, dry desert. But the state's southeast corner is blessed with abundant water-based recreation, especially at Bear Lake and Lava Hot Springs.

Bear Lake lies eighteen miles south of Montpelier on U.S. Highway 89. Not only is the water unbelievably blue; it also is home to several species of fish found nowhere else in the world, including the Bonneville Cisco. Fishing, camping, and boating are popular here. A national wildlife refuge on the lake's north end is home to deer, moose, and numerous waterfowl species. For more information, contact the Bear Lake Convention and Visitors Bureau at (208) 945-2072.

Lava Hot Springs was once a winter campground for the Bannock and Shoshone Indian tribes. White men discovered the site in 1812, and it became known as "Dempsey's Bath Tub." The springs lost their importance as an Indian camp after 1868, when tribal members were ordered to the Fort Hall Reservation. But Lava Hot Springs remains a popular gathering spot and is a growing retirement area.

A sea of green grass surrounds a huge, award-winning pool complex operated by the state of Idaho. Across town, another set of smaller pools maintain 110 degrees year-round. Several local hotels have their own private hot-water baths for guests, too. As if all this water isn't enough, the Portneuf River running through town provides plenty of trout-fishing and tubing action.

Special events include a major Corvette Car Show the last weekend in June and a mountain man rendezvous and "Pioneer Days" celebration in mid-July. Fall is another great time to visit, when the surrounding hillsides come alive in color. For more information, call the Lava Hot Springs Foundation at (208) 776-5221.

FORT HALL

Established in 1834 as a fur-trading post, **Fort Hall** later became an important resting stop for the emigrants. The post was originally situated fourteen miles north of Pocatello near what is now the shore of American Falls Reservoir, but the Bannock County centennial committee built a replica in Pocatello's Ross Park in 1963. To get there, follow the signs from Exit 67—the first Pocatello exit coming from the south—off of Interstate 15.

Actually, Fort Hall was the result of a grudge. Massachusetts native Nathaniel Wyeth originally wanted to start a trading post at the mouth of the Columbia River, but en route, he was convinced by fur traders Milton Sublette and Thomas Fitzpatrick to bring them $3,000 worth of goods they could sell at their Green River rendezvous the following year.

When Wyeth and his men returned the next spring, the Rocky Mountain Fur Company had dissolved and Wyeth was stuck with his wares. "Gentlemen," he reportedly told the traders, "I will yet roll a stone into your garden that you will never be able to get out." Wyeth built Fort Hall that summer, placing it on land he'd seen on earlier trips and naming it in honor of Henry Hall, the senior partner in the Boston firm that had financed his venture.

Like Jim Bridger, Wyeth became something of an absentee landlord. He was still interested in building a fort farther west, and he soon set off to pursue that idea. Eventually, however, he gave up and headed back east to pursue a career as an inventor. He sold Fort Hall to the Hudson's Bay Company in 1837 at a reported loss of $30,000. HBC set about improving the fort by encasing the log structure in adobe brick.

Despite the facelift, the reality of Fort Hall never quite matched up to the emigrants' expectations. One display in the replica museum notes that travelers often "wrote about seeing the whitewashed walls of the stockade glisten like a beacon in the distance. They also spoke of being disappointed by the roughness of the structure once they arrived." It's difficult to imagine the pioneers being let down by any fort when, after all, they had been on the road for many weeks with few signs of "civilization." Still, many of the pioneers were, after all, former urbanites whose notions of cities didn't quite jibe with the rough-and-ready settlements that passed for town life in the West.

After the British-based HBC bought the fort, emigrants were often convinced to abandon their plans to move to Oregon and head instead for California. In doing this, Hudson's Bay employees hoped to stem the tide of Americans flowing into the Northwest and preserve the region for their own country. Early parties that insisted on going to Oregon were talked into trading their wagons for pack trains since, the Hudson's Bay staff said, wagons couldn't stand the rugged terrain past this point.

But Marcus and Narcissa Whitman had already proved this conventional "wisdom" false. The missionary couple arrived here with their wagon in 1836. It was falling apart, but rather than switch to pack animals, Marcus Whitman converted the wagon to a cart and took it all the way to Fort Boise, nearly 300 miles away. Seven years later, Whitman passed this way again, leading the first great emigration to Oregon, a thousand people strong.

Exhibits at the Fort Hall replica include a blacksmith's shop, which lauds the blacksmith as an all-around craftsman, and a display on Indian lifestyles. Ask a staff member to run the videotape on Fort Hall's history.

The Fort Hall replica is open daily from 9 a.m. to 8 p.m. from June 1 through Sept. 15 and from 10 a.m. to 2 p.m. Tuesday through Saturday during April and May. Admission is $1 for adults, fifty cents ages 13 to 18, and twenty-five cents for ages 6 through 12. Ross Park also includes the Bannock County Historical Museum, a pool, rose garden, picnic

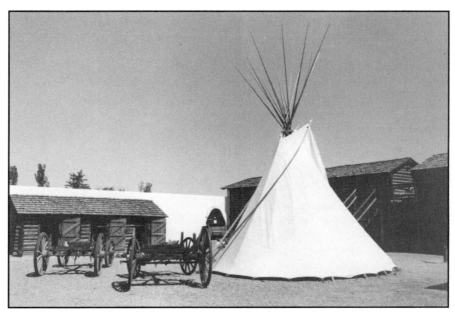

Fort Hall offers exhibits and replicas representing the fort's history and its influence on travelers along the Oregon Trail. Julie Fanselow photo.

areas, a playground, and a fenced field in which deer, antelope, elk, and bison roam. For more information, call (208) 234-1795.

After touring Fort Hall, spend a little time in Pocatello, Idaho's second-largest city with about 46,000 people. Long known as a railroad town and seat of higher learning (as home of Idaho State University), Pocatello also has an abundance of interesting historical buildings, including the Standrod House at 648 N. Garfield, usually considered the finest example of Victorian architecture in Idaho. A self-guiding architectural tour brochure is available at the Fort Hall replica. The Idaho Museum of Natural History on the ISU campus is another local favorite.

Pocatello offers a streetcar route that takes passengers to such places as Ross Park, the ISU campus, downtown, a golf course, and the town's two major malls. Fare is sixty cents, and the entire trip around town takes about an hour. For those looking for bed or board, Pocatello and its main suburb to the north, Chubbuck, offer wide selections of motels and restaurants.

The Fort Hall Indian Reservation north and west of Pocatello is home to more than 3,300 members of the Shoshone and Bannock tribes. The tribal government is headquartered at the town of Fort Hall, eight miles north of the junction of I-15 and I-86 near Pocatello. The Shoshone-Bannock Indian Festival and All-Indian Rodeos are held the second week of each August, and the tribes also operate a number of small businesses, including the Bannock Peak Truck Stop and Trading Post Complex at Exit 80 off of I-15. Browse here among Indian arts and crafts or eat at the Oregon Trail Restaurant, where the specialties include buffalo burgers, tacos, and fry bread. The city of Blackfoot, another ten miles north on I-15, is home of the Eastern Idaho State Fair, usually held in early September.

From Pocatello or points north, take I-15 to I-86 and continue west to Massacre Rocks State Park, twelve miles west of American Falls.

MASSACRE ROCKS

Most emigrant wagon trains that traversed southern Idaho encountered no trouble from the Indians. There were, however, occasional skirmishes. One such incident took place in August 1862, when ten emigrants and an unknown number of Indians were killed in two days of fighting. The battles painted this area with its unfairly harsh and gory name, **Massacre Rocks**.

During the trail era, the area was known as "Gate of Death" or "Devil's Gate," which referred to a narrow break in the rocks through which the wagon trains passed. (The natural gap disappeared in 1958 when rocks were blasted to construct Interstate 86.) Neither name is associated with the 1862 battles. In fact, those skirmishes took place east

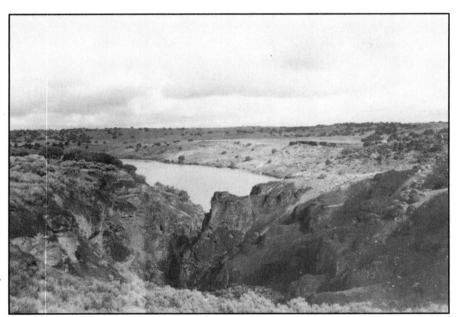

A skirmish between emigrants and Indians in 1862 gave Massacre Rocks its name. Julie Fanselow photo.

of the present-day state park. Local folks say it wasn't until the 1920s that the site became known as Massacre Rocks, but the name now seems stuck for good.

Happily, there is more to Massacre Rocks than historical hype. This state park has made the very most of its 900 acres, bounded on one side by the Snake River and on the other by I-86. Nearly seven miles of hiking trails offer the visitor close-up looks at everything from Oregon Trail remnants to more than 200 species of birds (including whistling swans, pelicans, blue herons, plus bald eagles in the winter); numerous desert plants (especially sagebrush, Utah juniper, and rabbit brush); and geological features.

Two trails in the area lead to a section of Oregon Trail ruts. Within the park, take the paved road to the parking area at its end. From there, follow the signs for the Oregon Trail. The trail to the ruts is 1.3 miles. The ruts may also be reached via the westbound rest area just past Exit 33 (Neeley Area) off of I-86. A trailhead at the rest area's west side leads to the Oregon Trail display. This route at 1.5 miles is a bit longer, but the rest area access may be more convenient for people who don't have much time to spend.

Massacre Rocks State Park has a small visitor center. Exhibits include the diary of Jane A. Gould, who traveled from Iowa to California in 1862 along the Oregon Trail and was in the area at the time of the skirmishes. Other facilities at the park include a campground with fully equipped restrooms, picnic areas, fishing access sites, and boat ramps. Nightly campfire programs take place each summer.

Idaho state parks charge a $2 per-vehicle entrance fee. For more information on Massacre Rocks, call (208) 548-2672.

American Falls Reservoir, just east of Massacre Rocks, is the largest reservoir on the Snake River and a favorite recreation spot for all of eastern Idaho. Fishing, boating, water skiing, and sailboarding are popular at the reservoir. The American Falls Marina offers camping, boat rentals, sailboarding lessons, and a dockside cafe.

West of Massacre Rocks, **Register Rock** was a major Oregon Trail campground. A shelter and fence guard a large basalt boulder on which visiting emigrants signed their names as early as 1849, and many of the signatures are still legible. Nearby, you can see where J.J. Hansen, a seven-year-old emigrant boy, carved an Indian's head on a smaller rock in 1866. Forty-seven years later, after he had become a professional sculptor, Hansen returned and dated the rock again.

Bonanza Bar, a gold camp, was established near here in 1878. Register Rock park offers picnic tables and shady relief from the Idaho desert. Register Road leads from the Massacre Rocks area past Register Rock and back to the interstate; there's no need to backtrack.

Once the pioneers crossed the Raft River, near what is now the small farming community of Yale, they faced what amounted to their last chance to decide on their final destination. Raft River marked the last jumping-off spot for the California Trail. Many emigrants reportedly didn't make up their mind until reaching this point!

Near Raft River, I-86 turns into I-84. Continue west on the interstate to Twin Falls, a good overnight stopping place, or detour via U.S. Highway 30 and see the BLM's fine **Milner Interpretive Area**. To do so, take Exit 208 off the interstate at Burley. Drive south over the Snake River and turn right on Bedke Boulevard. This road leads to U.S. Highway 30, which again parallels the trail. West of Burley, watch for signs pointing to the interpretive area, which also offers picnicking, camping, and boat access.

Although it was not an Oregon Trail site, Caldron Linn played a notable chapter in the history of western expansion. Near present-day Murtaugh, this was a narrow chute where the Snake River descended forty feet into a violent, churning pool. Wilson Price Hunt's party of Astorians traveled through the area in 1811 and had already lost a man and a canoe upstream when they came upon the swirling waters. Seeing no end to the torrent, they decided to abandon river travel.

Historical accounts differ as to whether Caldron Linn was known to emigrants on the Oregon Trail. But several artifacts including an ax head, beaver trap, and a musket stock from the Hunt expedition may be seen at the Idaho Historical Museum in Boise.

SIDETRIP: CITY OF ROCKS AND CRATERS OF THE MOON

The emigrants who turned southwest at Raft River soon came upon an amazing place not far from where Hudspeth's Cutoff joined the California Trail. Even in pioneer times, the area was known as the City of Rocks with its towering granite columns, some reaching sixty feet into the sky. Today, the City of Rocks is one of the nation's premier rock climbing sites, and its remoteness also attracts hikers, stargazers, photographers, sightseers, hunters, and campers.

One of the area's most famous attractions is (yet another) Register Rock, where emigrants wrote their names with axle grease. This is located at the first "Y" in the basin. Other notable formations include the Twin Sisters, Bath Rock, and Treasure Rock. These were all of great interest to the emigrants, and many described City of Rocks in their journals. Margaret Frink, who visited in July 1850, wrote this: "During the afternoon, we passed through a stone village composed of huge, isolated rocks of various and singular shapes, some resembling cottages, others steeples and domes. It is called City of Rocks, but I think the name Pyramid City more suitable. It is a sublime, strange and wonderful scene—one of nature's most interesting works."

To get to the City of Rocks, take Exit 216 off of I-84. Follow Idaho Highway 77 south to Connor. From Connor, take the Elba-Almo Highway to the City of Rocks. The last few miles are on unpaved road that is impassible in wet weather or during the spring runoff season. For more information, call the City of Rocks National Reserve at (208) 824-5519. The Albion Mountains en route to the City of Rocks are popular with hikers and hang-gliders.

After the Indian encounters of 1862, quite a few emigrants leaving Fort Hall took another trail alternate. This route, earlier used by fur traders, became known as Goodale's Cutoff after Timothy Goodale guided a large emigrant party across in 1862. But with its long fields of lava, Goodale's Cutoff was no easy road. J.C. Merrill wrote in 1864 that "at one place, we were obliged to drive over a huge rock just a little wider than the wagon. Had we gone a foot to the right or to the left, we would have rolled over."

Goodale's Cutoff passed near what is now one of Idaho's most fascinating natural areas, Craters of the Moon National Monument. Here, a strange and beautiful variety of lava flows and other volcanic features invite up-close inspection. Visitors can pitch a tent or park their trailer in a lava campground, hike to the top of a cinder cone, or explore an accessible section of officially designated wilderness. Most of the volcanic activity took place a mere 15,000 years ago, with eruptions occurring as recently as 2,000 years ago—a relative blip in geologic time.

Spring and fall are the best times to visit Craters of the Moon; summer is usually just too hot. In late May or early June, if the previous months have been wet enough, the black lava flows erupt with colorful wildflowers. Those who do visit during summer can beat the heat by exploring the Cave Area, a series of lava tubes. Wear sturdy shoes and bring a flashlight. For those seeking a quick tour, a seven-mile loop drive around the monument is an easy way to get acquainted with Craters' curiosities. Most of the hiking trails also begin on the loop road, and most are quite short.

Craters of the Moon is a considerable but delightful side trip from the Oregon Trail. The monument is eighteen miles west of Arco on U.S. Highway 93/26 and can be reached either by taking Highway 26 northwest from Blackfoot or Highway 93 northeast from Twin Falls. Either way, the monument is about 1.5 hours away. For more information on Craters of the Moon, call (208) 527-3257.

ROCK CREEK STAGE STATION

As increasing numbers of pioneers passed over the Oregon Trail, smart entrepreneurs saw opportunities to provide goods and services to the emigrants. One such man, James Bascom, built the **Rock Creek**

Stage Station southeast of Twin Falls in 1864. A year later, he added a log store, which still stands as the oldest building in south-central Idaho.

Rock Creek was a welcome sight to the emigrants, a good source of water and grass after a long, arid stretch across the Snake River Plain. The stage station also marked the intersection of the Oregon Trail, Ben Holladay's Overland Stage route, and the Kelton Road from Utah. For years, Rock Creek Station served as a popular emigrant campsite and transportation and commercial hub of south-central Idaho, much of which wasn't permanently settled until the late nineteenth century.

Soon after the stage station and store were built, the U.S. Army established Camp Reed to protect emigrants passing through the area. In 1875, Herman Stricker purchased the site. Today, visitors can still see the old log store, two stone cellars, and Stricker's 1900 home. One of the stone cellars served as the area's first jail, and a small cemetery nearby is said to contain the graves of three emigrants.

Rock Creek Station, also known as Stricker Ranch, can be reached by driving five miles south of Hansen, a small town along U.S. Highway 30, then one mile west. After visiting the ranch, consider driving on south into Rock Creek Canyon and the southernmost section of the Sawtooth National Forest. These "South Hills," as they're known locally, offer good camping, hiking, picnicking, and horseback riding.

Heading toward Twin Falls, consider a side trip to **Shoshone Falls**, well-marked by signs on Route 30. Although this 212-foot waterfall on the Snake River was five miles from the Oregon Trail, many travelers heard its roar and some hiked over to see the cascade for themselves. Shoshone Falls, sometimes called "the Niagara of the West," actually are thirty feet higher than Niagara Falls, but irrigation and hydropower demands have reduced the flow to a mere shadow of its former glory. Nevertheless, the city of Twin Falls maintains Shoshone Falls and adjacent Dierkes Lake as a park, and it is a popular spot for all kinds of outdoor fun.

Twin Falls itself, a city of about 29,000 people, is a community rooted in agriculture but growing as a regional retail and business center. This part of Idaho is known as the Magic Valley in honor of the irrigation projects that turned a desert into some of the world's most productive farmland. Located on the major north-south axis of U.S. Highway 93 and near I-84, Twin Falls accommodates a lot of tourist traffic, accounting for the city's unusually high density of motels and restaurants, most found along Blue Lakes Boulevard North and Addison Avenue West.

Much of Twin Falls' activity is concentrated around the College of Southern Idaho, a two-year school that serves as the region's educational and cultural capital. CSI's beautiful campus includes the Herrett Museum, with an outstanding collection of pre-Columbian artifacts and changing art exhibits. The Perrine Bridge spanning the Snake River north of Twin Falls is another top attraction, affording great views of the Snake

River Canyon. The canyon is home to two beautiful golf courses (Canyon Springs, reached via the south side, is public) and a new county park.

The area just north of the Perrine Bridge was traversed by the **Oregon Trail North Alternate**, which passed just a few hundred feet from the canyon rim. This undeveloped area offers the traveler a good idea of what the emigrants were experiencing as their wagons rolled across southern Idaho, often during the dog days of summer in 90- or 100-degree heat. John Fremont, who explored and mapped the West in the early 1840s, had this to say about what would become Idaho: "Water, though good and plenty, is difficult to reach as the river is hemmed in by high and vertical rocks and many of the streams are without water in the dry season. Grass is only to be found at the marked ramping places and barely sufficient to keep strong animals from starvation. Game, there is none. The road is very rough by volcanic rocks detrimental to wagons and carts. In sage bushes consists the only fuel. Lucky that by all these hardships the traveler is not harassed by the Indians, who are peaceable and harmless."

Visit the trail ruts by turning off Highway 93 into the BLM's Snake River Rim area and following the dirt roads east. From here, the curious can also get a good look at the ramp used by Evel Knievel in 1974 when he tried to leap the Snake River Canyon on a rocket-powered motorcycle.

A forty-five mile trip south from Twin Falls lands the wanderer in Nevada, where the border town of Jackpot offers gambling, semi-big-name entertainment, and great deals on food and lodging designed to lure visitors into the casinos. The formula is working: Parking lots in this town are filled with vehicles bearing license plates from as far afield as Alberta and Montana. Savvy Idahoans fill up on cheap food and skip the slots. In Twin Falls, The Sandpiper on Blue Lakes Boulevard is one of a handful of places offering live music. Downtown, talk is the main entertainment at Dunken's Draught House (which specializes in imported beers) and the Metropolis (which offers espresso and pastries). The Twin Falls Municipal Band, one of the nation's oldest, plays each Thursday evening during the summer at City Park on Shoshone Street near downtown.

Before they could leave what is now Twin Falls, the emigrants had to get across Rock Creek. This was no easy feat, for while the creek itself was only about twenty feet wide, the canyon walls were steep and rocky. The crossing was finally accomplished near what is now the Amalgamated Sugar Factory and the pioneers pushed westward.

From Twin Falls, the Oregon Trail stayed south of the Snake River. Modern travelers can, too, by taking Highway 30 (Addison Avenue) west out of town. This is the Thousand Springs Scenic Route, and it leads to the Hagerman Valley, one of Idaho's best-kept secrets.

SIDETRIP: SUN VALLEY/KETCHUM AND THE SAWTOOTH NATIONAL RECREATION AREA

In the 1930s, railroad executive Averell Harriman dispatched Austrian Count Felix Schaffgotsch to find the perfect American setting for a winter resort in the European tradition. The result was Sun Valley, America's first destination ski resort.

Since then, Sun Valley/Ketchum has remained a favorite playground of the rich and famous, largely because Idahoans, while friendly, tend to grant other folks their privacy. The resort towns also serve as gateway to the Sawtooth National Forest, Challis National Forest, and Sawtooth National Recreation Area, all of which offer abundant solitude and recreational possibilities.

Ketchum is the nerve center of the Sun Valley area. This small, cosmopolitan town offers lodging, nightlife, boutiques, art galleries, and sports-oriented shops where the young-at-heart can rent everything from mountain bikes to fly-fishing gear (and get free advice on where to play). The Sun Valley and Elkhorn resort complexes have their own selection of shopping, restaurants, and recreation. Whatever your sport, you are sure to find somewhere to enjoy it in the Sun Valley/Ketchum area, although prices can be steep for some activities. To economize, simply take advantage of the area's outstanding network of paved trails, all within gawking distance of Sun Valley's fabulous homes.

Sun Valley is best known for its skiing, but summer visitors can hoof it to the top of Baldy, its main mountain. From on top, hikers look across what seems like an endless vista of mountain ranges. Many other hiking opportunities can be found along Trail Creek Road east of Sun Valley and Highway 75 north of Ketchum.

Ernest Hemingway spent his last years in Ketchum, and a memorial to the author sits along Trail Creek just northeast of the Sun Valley golf course (on the right side of Trail Creek Road). Visitors can also see "Papa's" grave in the Ketchum cemetery, or cast a line into Silver Creek, one of his favorite fishing spots.

North of Ketchum, Highway 75 winds into the Sawtooth National Recreation Area. A visitor center about eight miles north of Ketchum has information on trails and other opportunities, as well as free auto-tape tours which can be borrowed and played to describe the area's features and history. North of the visitor center, the highway soon climbs to the top of Galena Summit. A turnout just past the summit has a great panoramic view of the Sawtooth Mountains and the headwaters of the Salmon River. Most folks would say the heart of the SNRA is Redfish Lake. Situated at the base of the Sawtooths near the town of Stanley, Redfish is a beloved site for hiking (try the Bench Lakes trail on the west side), boating, camping, and horseback riding.

The town of Stanley is known for its lively summer nightlife and several special events, including the Sawtooth Mountain Mama Arts and

Crafts Fair, usually held the third week of July. Northeast of Stanley, Highway 75 becomes the Salmon River Scenic Route. Attractions along this stretch include whitewater rafting, fishing, camping, and soaking at Sunbeam hot springs. Also consider a visit to the Land of the Yankee Fork State Park, including the old gold towns of Custer and Bonanza.

Ketchum/Sun Valley is eighty-four miles north of Twin Falls, and Stanley is another sixty miles northwest. For more information on Sun Valley/Ketchum, contact the Chamber of Commerce at (800) 634-3347. The Stanley Chamber of Commerce may be reached at (208) 664-3411, and the Sawtooth National Recreation Area's phone number is (208) 726-SNRA.

THOUSAND SPRINGS

Eighteen miles past the Rock Creek crossing, the trail returned to the Snake River at Kanaka Rapids. The rapids were also known as **Fremont's Fishing Falls**, after John Fremont publicized them following his 1843 exploration. Here, the pioneers traded with Indians, for whom this was an important salmon fishery.

West of Twin Falls, Highway 30 stays out of sight of the river through the towns of Filer and Buhl. Filer is home of the Twin Falls

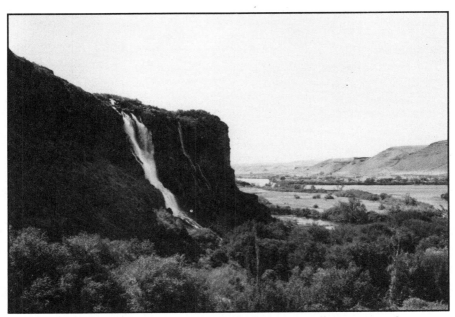

Water gushes from the black volcanic rock that forms the cliff walls above the Snake River at Thousand Springs. Julie Fanselow photo.

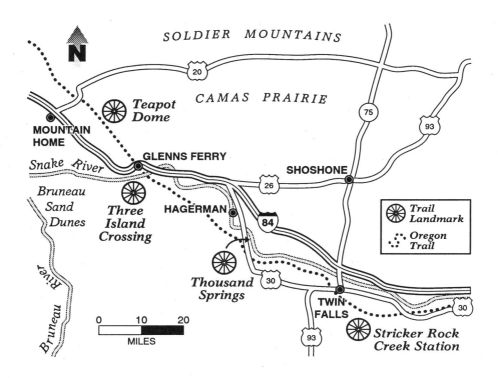

County Fair and Rodeo, held early each September, and Buhl boasts the world's largest commercial trout farm, Clear Springs. Past Buhl, the road zigzags north, then east, the north again, all the while getting closer to the canyon. After a few final descending bends, the **Thousand Springs** are in view. And although there are far fewer springs today than in emigrant times, the white water gushing from the black canyon walls is as enchanting as ever.

Where does the water come from? Some originates in eastern Idaho, where the Big Lost River and several other waterways abruptly sink into the ground. From there, the water moves ever so slowly—possibly just ten feet a day—through the underground Snake River aquifer, one of the largest groundwater systems in the world. Rain, snow melt, and irrigation runoff add to the aquifer before the springs finally burst forth into the canyon.

In 1911, an Arizona company built a 400-foot long flume along the north canyon wall to capture the water and produce electricity. At one time, the Thousand Springs plant produced about twenty percent of Idaho Power's electric load. Today, however, the plant's output fills a far smaller fraction of the utility's demands. There is talk of dismantling the plant and letting the springs flow free once again, but no one's laying good odds it will ever happen.

Around 1852, a road on the north side of the Snake River came into use. Some emigrants who decided to cross forded the river, but most used a ferry. After years of service to emigrant and local traffic, Payne's Ferry broke away and sank three miles downstream. Present-day Hagerman also was the site of Camp Reed No. 2, another temporary military post established to protect pioneer traffic.

Minnie Miller, a Utah businesswoman, owned an island in the Snake River during much of the first half of the 20th century and used it to develop one of the nation's top Guernsey cattle herds. Today, the land is owned by The Nature Conservancy, which offers tours in conjunction with nearby Malad Gorge State Park on Saturday mornings during the summer. Most tours are free, but several have special themes (including the Oregon Trail) and conclude with a lunch and wine tasting for $10. Call (208) 837-4505 for more information and directions to the preserve, which must be accessed via the canyon's north side.

The Thousand Springs signal entry into the Hagerman Valley. Hagerman consistently posts the highest temperatures in Idaho, and the mild year-round climate attracts recreationists and retirees. Top attractions include several commercial hot springs, some with private baths, and a number of good fishing holes (try the Oster Lakes, Anderson Ponds, or Billingsley Creek). Visitors can tour a winery, Rose Creek; see artists in action at the Snake River Pottery west of town on the old Bliss Grade; or take a float trip down the Snake River.

The nearby Hagerman fossil beds were discovered by a local farmer in 1928. The Smithsonian Institute conducted several expeditions to the site and unearthed 130 skulls and fifteen skeletons of an early, zebra-like horse. Other fossils found here preserved early forms of camel, peccary, beaver, turtle, and freshwater fish. The Hagerman Valley Historical Museum at 100 S. State St. features a Smithsonian model of the prehistoric horse. The fossil beds themselves are now a national monument, but the site remains largely uninterpreted and inaccessible to tourists.

West of Thousand Springs, the emigrants found another good site for trading with the Indians at **Upper Salmon Falls**. Writing of the area's beauty, Fremont called it "one of those places that the traveler turns again and again to fix in his memory." Highway 30 climbs out of the Hagerman Valley to Bliss, a small community near I-84. From Bliss, a seven-mile backtrack east on I-84 to the Tuttle exit leads to Malad Gorge State Park, another site on the Oregon Trail North Alternate. Park staff here found remnants of the emigrant trail while cleaning up a local garbage dump a few years ago. A short path leads from a parking lot to the deep, scenic gorge over the Malad River, which at just 2.5 miles long has sometimes been called the world's shortest river.

From Bliss, continue west on I-84 to Glenns Ferry, site of one of the Oregon Trail's toughest river crossings.

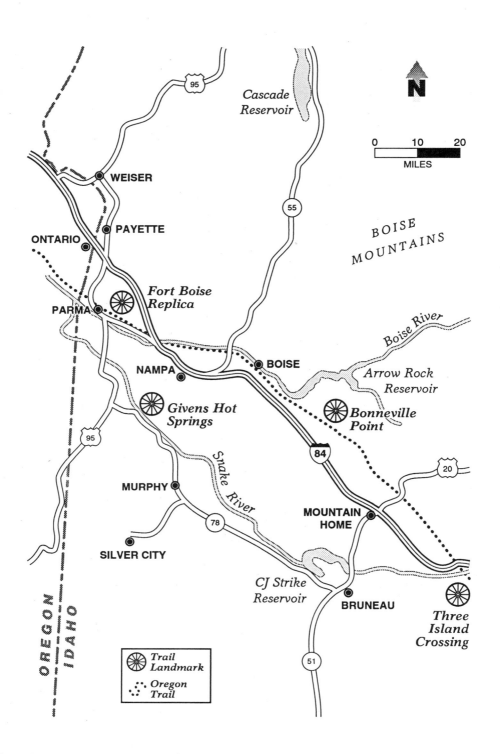

THREE ISLAND CROSSING

Near present-day Glenns Ferry, the emigrants faced another difficult choice. They could attempt the **Three Island Crossing** to a shorter, easier route north of the Snake River, or they could stay on the dry, rough Oregon Trail South Alternate.

Crossing the river meant contending with its formidable width, deep channels, and swift currents, but about half the emigrants decided to try. Today, the site is part of Three Island Crossing State Park, where a re-enactment staged the second Saturday each August features exact replicas of wagons, pack trains, and period clothing.

History shows that the emigrants actually used two different routes to cross the river here. One crossing that could be made without swimming or floating was called Three Island Ford. Two Island Crossing, one mile upstream, was more difficult and dangerous because wagons had to be floated across the Snake. (This crossing actually has three islands in sight, but only the southernmost and middle islands were used.) Most emigrants believed these separate crossings were the same, which is how the area became known as Three Island Crossing.

Crossing the river took considerable preparation and time. Men would swim to the opposite side of the river then use ropes to pull the wagons across. Wagons and carts often capsized; livestock sometimes drowned. Few emigrants who passed here failed to mention the crossing in their diaries. P.V. Crawford, who emigrated in 1851, said the ordeal took the better part of three days. On July 31, he wrote: "This day we spent in arranging for and crossing the river. We accomplished this by corking two wagons and lashing them together. By this means we were able to ferry over a wagon and its load at each trip. By noon we had our boat ready and began operations, but found it slow business, but succeeded in getting over safely, but not the same day, for we had to lay by on account of wind. Leaving part of our camping on each side of the river, here we had both sides to guard."

Narcissa Whitman gave a detailed description of her party's crossing, which included loading packs atop the tallest horses in an effort to keep possessions dry. "Husband had considerable difficulty in crossing the cart," she wrote. "Both cart and mules were turned upside down in the river and entangled in the harness. The mules would have drowned but for a desperate struggle to get them ashore. Then after putting two of the strongest horses before the cart, and two men swimming behind to steady it, they succeeded in getting it across. I once thought that crossing streams would be the most dreaded part of the journey. I can now cross the most difficult stream without the least fear." The Three Island Crossing passed into history in 1869 when Gus P. Glenn established a ferry a short distance above the crossing.

Three Island State Park is reached via Exit 120 off of I-84. Drive south into Glenns Ferry and follow the signs to the park. From the bank of the Snake River here, visitors can see the islands used in the crossing as well as scars worn by wagon wheels on the river's south side.

The park's visitor center features several historical displays including a large map of all emigrant trails in Idaho. And for those who haven't had a chance to see bison on your trip so far, here's an opportunity. The state park has its own herd, donated from the National Bison Range at Moiese, Montana. The shaggy beasts now live in an enclosed pasture in the park's southeast corner, along with longhorn cattle that were brought to Idaho as a gift from the State of Oklahoma. Other activities at the park include camping, swimming, fishing, and picnicking. The Oregon Trail Mountain Bike Tour starts here one Saturday each spring. Call Three Island State Park at (208) 366-2394 for more information.

Glenns Ferry has limited visitor services: a couple of cafes, one small motel, and an RV park. Mountain Home, another thirty-five miles west on I-84, is the next major town, and it offers a wider range of lodging and restaurants. From Mountain Home, it's about a half-hour drive to Bonneville Point, which marked the end of the emigrants' trek through the great Idaho desert.

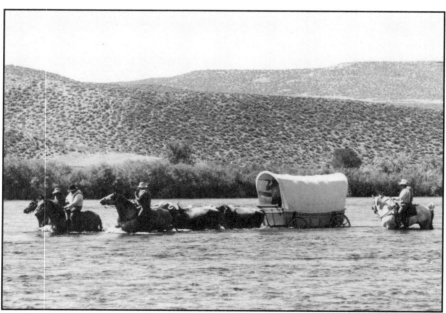

This re-enactment of the Three Island Crossing looks tame compared to tales told by emigrants. Julie Fanselow photo.

SIDETRIP: SOUTHWEST IDAHO'S RIVER AND CANYON COUNTRY

For some, the Three Island Crossing proved too much. Cornelia A. Sharp, an 1852 emigrant, wrote on Aug. 9 that her party "made several attempts to swim our cattle, but without success." The next day, they "abandoned the idea of crossing the river; gathered up our cattle, hitched up our teams and took the sand and sage for it."

The South Alternate was a rough road but it did offer some spectacular scenery, including sand dunes, canyons, rivers, and buttes. About forty miles west of Glenns Ferry and reachable today via Idaho Highway 78 from Exit 112 or 114 off of I-84, Bruneau Dunes State Park boasts the tallest sand dunes in North America, the largest rising 470 feet from the ground. The state park offers excellent fishing, camping, and hiking. The Big Dune hike is an unforgettable experience, but it's best tackled early in the day before the sun gets too hot. Call (208) 366-7919 for more information.

After passing the sand dunes, the wagon trains rolled on toward the Bruneau River. Today's Bruneau Canyon is home to bighorn sheep and pronghorn antelope, and it may be viewed by hanging a left at the small town of Bruneau then traveling eighteen miles southeast on the signed road. The Bruneau, Owyhee, and Jarbidge rivers, all in this area, feature scenic whitewater rafting through some of the most remote areas of America. Call the Idaho Outfitters and Guides Association at (208) 342-1438 for information on rafting, hunting, and packing trips in the region.

Highway 78 west of Bruneau continues to parallel the South Alternate. C.J. Strike Reservoir harbors fine boating, water skiing, fishing, and camping. The Snake River Birds of Prey Natural Area stretches from Grandview to Murphy; see this book's Boise section for more information. Murphy, seat of vast Owyhee County, is possibly the nation's smallest county seat. It has just one general store, one parking meter (placed in front of the courthouse as a prank), and maybe fifty people. There are only about 8,500 people in all of Owyhee County, which at 7,643 square miles is bigger than New Jersey.

The worst tragedy on the Oregon Trail happened in this area, near Castle Creek about midway between Grandview and Murphy. During September 1860, the Elijah Otter (or Utter) party consisting of forty-four people, eight wagons, and more than fifty head of livestock, had a battle with more than 100 Indians. During the fight, eleven emigrants and some twenty-five Indians were slain. Of the thirty-three emigrants who survived the battle, seventeen died or were killed soon after. This was the largest recorded confrontation between whites and Indians at any place along the trail.

Oregon-bound emigrants often stopped at what is now Givens Hot Springs to wash their clothes and camp. One traveler said the springs were "sufficiently hot to boil eggs." Milford and Martha Givens had seen the springs on their way west and later decided to return and settle in the area. Today, Givens Hot Springs remains in the family and is a popular place for soaking, swimming, and camping.

Toward the end of the Oregon Trail era, mining became big business throughout southwestern Idaho. Silver City was one of the territory's busiest boom towns. In fact, at one time the silver production from its more than 250 mines was surpassed only by the Comstock Lode in Nevada. Silver City remains home to just a few dozen people, but many buildings remain standing with only minimal commercial activity to detract from the near-ghost town ambience. To visit Silver City, take the Silver City Road five miles southeast of Murphy. The twenty-three mile unimproved road takes about an hour to drive. It's rough going, but most vehicles can make it.

BONNEVILLE POINT

At **Bonneville Point**, the pioneers found a welcome sight that marked the end of their difficult trip across Idaho's dry and dusty plains. Captain B.L.E. Bonneville's party arrived here in May 1833 and, seeing the verdant valley below, called out "Les Bois, les bois, voyes les bois!" ("The trees, the trees, look at the trees!") For years afterward, this spot continued to delight weary emigrants. "When we arrived at the top we got a grand view of the Boise River Valley," Cecilia E. M. Adams wrote. "It is filled or covered with dry grass and a few trees immediately along the bank, the first we have seen in more than a month." Fremont wrote of his delight at the Boise River, "a beautiful rapid stream, with clear mountain water" and said he was "delighted this afternoon to make a pleasant camp under fine old trees again."

Bonneville Point was about 1,450 miles from the trailhead in Independence. The emigrants had now completed about three-quarters of their journey. This—combined with the valley view—was cause to celebrate, even though some rough terrain still lie ahead. "You doubtless will think I regret taking this long and tiresome trip," Elizabeth Wood wrote in August 1851, "But no, I have a great desire to see Oregon."

To reach Bonneville Point, take Exit 64 off of I-84 and follow the signs north. The BLM has erected an interpretive kiosk, and a long stretch of excellent wagon ruts may be seen nearby. Bonneville Point also lies along a proposed BLM scenic byway that will guide modern travelers through an area which has an especially high concentration of still-visible trail remnants. It isn't certain how soon interpretive signs will be posted, but more information on the route is available from the BLM's Boise District Office, 3948 Development Avenue, Boise, ID 83705. The phone number is (208) 384-3300.

From Bonneville Point, the wagon trains rolled into the valley, just south of what is now Lucky Peak Reservoir, a popular recreation area. In

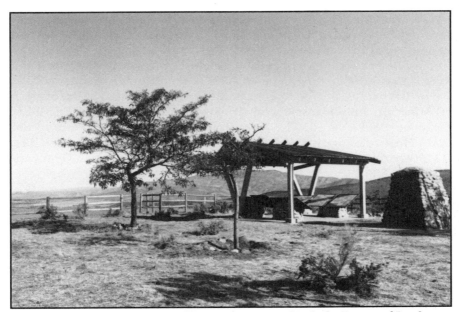

Excellent wagon ruts can be seen from the interpretive kiosk the Bureau of Land Management erected at Bonneville Point. Julie Fanselow photo.

1863, an Army calvary post called **Fort Boise** was built to protect both the emigrants and gold miners who were flooding into the region. The city of Boise grew up around the fort, and the community became an important stop during later years of travel on the Oregon Trail. The fort was deactivated in 1913, but several buildings are still in use as a Veterans Administration medical center. An old cemetery with about 200 graves dating back to the 1860s and 1870s is behind the medical center. A city park is nearby.

Another Fort Boise was built much earlier by the Hudson's Bay Company about five miles northwest of present-day Parma. Nothing remains of the original fort, but a replica may be seen in a Parma park.

SIDETRIP: BOISE ATTRACTIONS

Survey after recent survey has dubbed Idaho's capital city, Boise, as one of the nation's most desirable places to live. The rapid recent growth has meant big increases in traffic, real estate prices, and espresso carts. Yet despite the urbanization, Boise—with a metropolitan-area population of about 180,000—retains a lot of small-town charm and friendliness. Throw in a four-year university and recreation opportunities galore, and it's easy to understand why Boise is booming.

For the visitor, many top attractions are found in a surprisingly compact area between the state capitol and Boise State University. The thirteen-mile Boise River Greenbelt welcomes cyclists, joggers, power walkers, in-line skaters, and just-plain strollers, while tubers often float the river. (Bikes, skates, tubes, and rafts can be rented near the river.) Julia Davis Park includes a zoo, the Boise Art Museum, and the Idaho Historical Museum, with its fascinating displays on the Oregon Trail and other aspects of Idaho's past. The Boise Tour Train also departs from Julia Davis Park, offering citywide views from an 1890s-style locomotive. The Discovery Center of Idaho, in the same vicinity, features hands-on educational exhibits for children and adults.

Boise's summer is full of special events. The Idaho Shakespeare Festival performs in open-air theater at Park Center. The Boise River Festival, started in the early 1990s, has already become one of Idaho's major annual events. Held late each June, it features a nighttime river parade with lighted floats. The Western Idaho Fair in nearby Garden City runs the end of each August with big-name entertainment and carnival rides. Once college football season starts, the BSU Broncos play in what may be the world's only stadium with blue artificial turf.

In providing entertainment, Boise hasn't quite caught up with its growing population. Big-name pop and country concerts are still fairly rare, but when they hit town, most acts play at the BSU Pavillion. Go to The Flicks at Sixth and Myrtle for the latest in international and independent films and an adjacent cafe. Les Bois Park features parimutuel horse racing each May through August.

The World Birds of Prey Center, located on a bluff south of Boise off of South Cole Road, helps breed and preserve a variety of endangered species of birds. Spring visitors may have the chance to see newly hatched peregrine falcons and eagles. The facility may be toured by appointment only; call (208) 362-3716 for information. The Snake River Birds of Prey Natural Area is best approached via Highway 69 south of Kuna. (Allow an hour one-way for the trip.) It is home to the largest concentration of nesting eagles, hawks, and prairie falcons on earth. View the area from the rim or take a guided boat trip from Swan Falls Dam. For more information, call (208) 334-1582.

During the 1860s, more gold was mined from the mountains northeast of Boise than from all of Alaska. Idaho City, twenty-two miles from Boise via Idaho Highway 21, was once the largest city in the Northwest and a wild mining town to boot. Legend has it that only twenty-eight of the 200 people buried in the town's Boot Hill died a natural death. Idaho City today is heavily tourist-oriented, with five restaurants and a couple of small motels. The neighboring Boise National Forest is full of great mountain vistas and campgrounds.

For more information on Boise-area attractions, contact the Boise Convention and Visitors Bureau at (800) 635-5240.

FORT BOISE

The Hudson's Bay Company built Fort Boise in 1834, partially in retaliation for the American presence Nathaniel Wyeth had erected at Fort Hall. Fort Boise was situated on the east bank of the Snake River about eight miles north of the mouth of the Boise River. Although it was built as a fur trading post, Fort Boise soon switched its emphasis to serving the emigrants, and it was a welcome outpost after 300 miles of dry travel from Fort Hall.

Fort Boise was managed for its first decade by Francois Payette, a successful French-Canadian fur trapper. Payette was well-liked by the emigrants; one visitor described him as "exceedingly polite, courteous, and hospitable." An 1845 report on the post spoke of "two acres under cultivation...1,991 sheep, seventy-three pigs, seventeen horses, and twenty-seven meat cattle." But when the emigrants started to arrive, they would sometimes completely deplete the fort's stores of flour, tea, coffee, and other staples.

Fort Boise was the jumping-off point for an especially ill-conceived trail cutoff. Stephen H.L. Meek, leading an 1845 emigrant party headed by Capt. Elijah White, convinced many of its members to join him in trying a new way to the Willamette—a route that would avoid the Blue Mountains but which had never been traveled by wagons before. Historians say even Meek probably didn't know the way, but between 150 and 200 wagons followed him anyway, possibly thinking that Meek was as smart as his brother, Joe, one of the West's best guides.

It was a big mistake. The route along the Malheur River offered little grass for the livestock, and it was murder on the animals' feet. The emigrants sometimes went days without water. Fever struck the party and some children died. To top it all off, the travelers were lost, and Meek finally had to go on ahead to find a rescue party. Writing in *The Oregon Trail Revisited*, Gregory Franzwa noted that was probably a good idea on Meek's part— "the thoroughly disillusioned emigrants would have blown his brains out had he stayed in camp another day."

Meek found a knowledgeable mountain man named Black Harris at the Columbia River, and Harris agreed to lead the rescue. He found the starving pioneers near the mouth of Tygh Creek and led them down the Deschutes River to the Columbia and to safety. Of nearly 500 who started out with Meek, more than seventy-five people had died.

In 1853, flooding extensively damaged Fort Boise, and historians indicate that attempts to rebuild—if any—were probably futile due to mounting tensions with the Indians. Troubles in the area culminated with the Ward Massacre, in which eighteen emigrants (out of a party of twenty) died. Hudson's Bay Company abandoned Fort Boise two years later. Today, the land serves as a state wildlife management area. No signs of the fort remain, but its approximate location is marked by a striking, British-influenced monument that features a stately lion's head atop a pedestal.

The people of Parma have built a Fort Boise replica in their town, five miles southeast of the original fort site. It is open only from 1 to 3 p.m. Fridays, Saturdays and Sundays during June, July, and August, but to see it during off-hours, call the Parma City Hall at (208) 722-5138 to make arrangements. Parma also celebrates its role in trail history late each May with the Old Fort Boise Days celebration.

The replica was built to the old fort's exact dimensions, although cosmetic changes were made to accommodate modern building codes. In addition to the emigrant story, the Fort Boise Replica has artifacts and displays from later years in which southwest Idaho was permanently settled. One room features a desk built in 1891 by a boy whose family was traveling to Oregon when their money ran out and they decided to stay. Another exhibit tells how Parma is the only Idaho town to have produced two of the state's governors: Clarence Baldridge, a Republican, and Ben Ross, a Democrat. Visitors may also view a video on Fort Boise history.

A statue and historical marker on the replica lawn tell the story of Marie Dorian, an Iowa Indian who came to the area with Wilson Price Hunt's party of Astorians in 1811. (Dorian had, in fact, excused herself briefly on that trip to give birth to a boy somewhere near present-day North Powder, Oregon.) Three years later, Marie and her two children were the sole survivors of a mid-January battle with Bannock Indians at a nearby fur-trading post. They set out with two horses on a two-hundred-mile retreat through deep snow and were finally rescued by a Columbia River band of Walla Walla Indians in April.

The park adjacent to the fort replica includes a small campground with showers and a dump station, as well as shady picnic spots and a playground. To get to Parma, leave I-84 at Exit 26, drive south over the interstate and follow U.S. Highway 20/26 to Parma, thirteen miles northwest.

Near Old Fort Boise, the emigrants crossed the Snake River and entered what is now Oregon. Modern travelers can continue west via I-84 or U.S. Highway 26, which enters Oregon near Vale and Keeney Pass.

LODGING

MONTPELIER, IDAHO

Best Western Crest Motel, (800) 528-1234, 243 N. 4th St., $47-$50.

Budget Motel, (208) 847-1273, 240 N. 4th St., $20-$40.

Michelle Motel, (208) 847-1772, 401 Boise St., $28.

Park Motel, (208) 847-1911, 745 Washington, $27.

SODA SPRINGS, IDAHO

Caribou Lodge and Motel, (208) 547-3377, 110 W. 2nd S., $25-$43.

J-R Inn, (208) 547-3366, 179 W. 2nd S., $32.

Lakeview Motel, (208) 547-4351, 341 W. 2nd S., $22-$40.

LAVA HOT SPRINGS, IDAHO

Home Hotel and Motel, (208) 776-5507, 305 Emerson, $21-$31.

Lava Ranch Inn Motel, (208) 776-9917, 9611 Highway 30.

Lava Spa and Tumbling Waters Motel, (208) 776-5589, 359 E. Main, $30-$65.

Oregon Trail Motel, (208) 776-5000, 119 E. Main, $25-$35.

Riverside Inn & Hot Springs, (800) 733-5504, 255 Portneuf, $40-$75.

Royal Hotel Bed & Breakfast, (208) 776-5216, 11 E. Main, $31-$59.

POCATELLO, IDAHO

Best Western Cotton Tree Inn, (800) 528-1234, 1415 Bench Road, $54-$74.

Best Western Weston Inn, (800) 528-1234, 745 S. 5th Ave., $36.

Days Inn, (800) 325-2525, 133 W. Burnside, $45.

Howard Johnson Hotel, (800) IGO-HOJO, 1399 Bench Road, $65.

Motel 6, (208) 237-7880, 291 W. Burnside, $21-$39.

Oxbow Motor Inn, (208) 237-3100, 4333 Yellowstone, $25-$39.

Pocatello Quality Inn, (800) 638-7949, 1555 Pocatello Creek Road, $52-$62.

Sundial Inn, (208) 233-0451, 835 S. 5th St., $32.

Thunderbird Motel, (208) 232-6330, 1415 S. 5th Ave., $24-$27.

AMERICAN FALLS, IDAHO

Hillview Motel, (208) 226-5151, I-86 Exit 40, $30.

Ronnez Motel, (208) 226-9658, 411 Lincoln, $23-$40.

RUPERT, IDAHO

Flamingo Lodge Motel, (208) 436-4321, Highway 25, $25-$45.

Uptown Motel, (208) 436-4036, Highway 24, $22-$35.

BURLEY, IDAHO

Best Western Burley Inn, (800) 528-1234, 800 N. Overland Ave., $48.

Budget Motel, (800) 635-4952, 900 N. Overland Ave., $38.

Greenwell Motel, (208) 678-5576, 904 E. Main, $28-$36.

Parish Motel, (208) 678-5505, 721 E. Main, $19-$35.

TWIN FALLS, IDAHO

Amber Inn Motel, (208) 825-5200, I-84 Exit 182.

AmeriTel Inn, (208) 736-8000, 1377 Blue Lakes Blvd. N.

Best Western Apollo Motor Inn, (800) 528-1234, 296 Addison Ave. W., $41.

Best Western Canyon Springs Inn, (800) 528-1234, 1357 Blue Lakes Blvd. N., $53-$58.

EconoLodge, (800) 446-6900, 320 Main Ave. S., $29-$36.

Monterey Motor Inn, (208) 733-5151, 433 Addison Ave. W., $32.

Motel 6, (208) 734-3993, 1472 Blue Lakes Blvd. N., $27-$45.

Super 8 Motel, (800) 843-1991, 1261 Blue Lakes Blvd. N., $42.

Weston Plaza Hotel, (800) 333-7829, 1350 Blue Lakes Blvd. N., $47-$56.

BUHL, IDAHO

Oregon Trail Motel, (208) 543-8814, 510 S. Broadway (Highway 30), $36.

Siesta Motel, (208) 543-6427, 629 S. Broadway, $24-$35.

HAGERMAN, IDAHO

Hagerman Valley Inn, (208) 837-6196, State and Hagerman streets, $34.

Rock Lodge Resort, (208) 837-4822, 17940 Highway 30.

Sportsman's River Resort, (208) 837-6364, south of town on Highway 30, $20-$35.

BLISS, IDAHO

Amber Inn, (208) 352-4441, I-84 Exit 141, $26-$30.

GLENNS FERRY, IDAHO

Redford Motel, (208) 366-2421, I-84 Exit 120, $19-$50.

MOUNTAIN HOME, IDAHO

Best Western Foothills Motor Inn, (800) 528-1234, 1080 Highway 20, $43-$60.

Hi Lander Motel, (208) 587-3311, 615 S. 3rd W., $29-$34.

Motel Thunderbird, (208) 587-7927, 910 Sunset Strip (Highway 30), $25-$28.

Sleep Inn, (800) 4CHOICE, 1180 Highway 20, $44.

Towne Center Motel, (208) 587-3373, 410 N. 2nd E., $28-$33.

BOISE, IDAHO

Best Western Safari Motor Inn, (800) 541-6651, 1070 Grove St., $41-$46.

The Boisean Motel, (800) 365-3645, 1300 S. Capitol Blvd., $41-$59.

Capri Motel, (208) 344-8617, 2600 Fairview, $25-$40.

Comfort Inn, (800) 4CHOICE, 2526 Airport Way, $43-$38.

Holiday Inn, (800) HOLIDAY, 3300 Vista Ave., $47-$70.

Idaho Heritage Inn Bed & Breakfast, (208) 342-8066, 109 W. Idaho, $55-$80.

Idanha Hotel, (208) 342-3611, 928 Main St.

Nendels Inn, (208) 344-4030, 2155 N. Garden, $38-$46.

Red Lion Hotel Downtowner, (800) 547-8010, 1800 Fairview, $54-$94.

Rodeway Inn, (800) 228-2000, 1115 N. Curtis Road, $55-$63.

Shilo Inn Boise Airport, (800) 222-2244, 4111 Broadway, $55-$67.

University Inn, (208) 345-7170, 2360 University Dr., $47-$51.

MERIDIAN, IDAHO

Knotty Pine Motel, (208) 888-2727, 1423 E. 1st St., $25-$45.

NAMPA, IDAHO

Desert Inn, (208) 467-1161, 115 9th Ave. S., $34-$48.

Five Crowns Inn, (208) 466-3594, 908 3rd St. S., $34.

Shilo Inn Nampa Suites, (800) 222-2244, 1401 Shilo Drive, $49-$65.

Super 8 Motel, (800) 843-1991, 624 Nampa Blvd., $31-$52.

Starlite Motel, (208) 466-9244, 320 11th Ave. N., $23-$40.

CALDWELL, IDAHO

Comfort Inn, (800) 4CHOICE, 901 Specht Ave., $50.

Holiday Motel, (208) 454-3888, 512 Frontage Road, $24-$50.

Manning House Bed & Breakfast, (208) 459-7899, 1803 S. 10th Ave., $35-$45.

Sundowner Motel, (208) 459-1585, 1002 Arthur, $36-$38.

PARMA, IDAHO

Court Motel, (208) 722-5579, 712 Grove St., $25-$40.

PAYETTE, IDAHO

Montclair Motel, (208) 642-2693, 625 S. Main, $20-$40.

CAMPING

MONTPELIER, IDAHO

Bear Lake State Park, (208) 945-2790, twenty miles south on Highway 89; follow signs.

Montpelier KOA, (208) 847-0863, two miles east on Highway 89.

SODA SPRINGS, IDAHO

Dike Lake, (208) 529-1020, eleven miles north on Highway 34. Primitive sites.

LAVA HOT SPRINGS, IDAHO

Cottonwood Family Campground, (208) 776-5295, Highway 30.

Lava Mobile Estates and Campground, (208) 776-5447.

Lava Ranch Inn RV Camping, (208) 776-9917, 9611 Highway 30.

POCATELLO, IDAHO

Pocatello KOA, (208) 233-6851, 9815 Pocatello Creek Road.

AMERICAN FALLS, IDAHO

Indian Springs, (208) 226-2174, three miles west on Highway 37.

Massacre Rocks State Park, (208) 548-2672, ten miles west on I-86.

BURLEY, IDAHO

Snake River Campground, (208) 654-2133, I-84 Exit 216.

HAZELTON, IDAHO

Greenwood RV Park, (208) 829-5735, I-84 Exit 194.

TWIN FALLS, IDAHO

Anderson Campground, (208) 733-6756, I-84 Exit 182.

Nat-Soo-Pah Hot Springs & RV Park, (208) 655-4337, sixteen miles south on Highway 93; follow signs.

Twin Falls-Jerome KOA, (208) 324-4169, I-84 Exit 173. Kamping Kabins.

Several Forest Service campgrounds are located in the Sawtooth National Forest south of Twin Falls. Call (208) 737-3200 for information.

HAGERMAN, IDAHO

Banbury Hot Springs, (208) 543-4098, south of town off Highway 30.

Miracle Hot Springs, (208) 543-6002, south of town on Highway 30.

Rock Lodge and Creekside RV Park, (208) 837-4822, one mile north on Highway 30.

Sligar's 1000 Springs, (208) 837-4987, south of town on Highway 30.

Sportsman's River Resort, (208) 837-6364, six miles south on Highway 30.

GLENNS FERRY, IDAHO

Three Island Crossing State Park, (208) 366-2394, I-84 Exit 120; follow signs.

Trails West RV Park, (208) 366-2002.

MOUNTAIN HOME, IDAHO

Bruneau Dunes State Park, (208) 366-7919, eighteen miles south on Highway 51; two miles east on Highway 78.

Golden Rule KOA, (208) 587-5111, 220 E. 10th N.

BOISE, IDAHO

Americana Kampground, (208) 344-5733, 3600 Americana Terrace.

Boise KOA, (208) 345-7673, I-84 Exit 57. Kamping Kabins.

Fiesta RV Park, (208) 375-8207, 11101 Fairview Ave.

On the River RV Park, (208) 375-7432, 6000 Glenwood.

Several Forest Service campgrounds are located in the Boise National Forest near Boise. Call (208) 364-4100 for information.

MARSING, IDAHO

Givens Hot Springs, (208) 495-2437, eleven miles southeast on Highway 78.

CALDWELL, IDAHO

Aspen Village, (208) 454-0553, I-84 Exit 26.

Camp Caldwell Campground, (208) 454-0279, I-84 Exit 26.

PARMA, IDAHO

Old Fort Boise Park, (208) 722-5138, city park along Highway 20/26.

FRUITLAND, IDAHO

Curtis' Neat Retreat, (208) 452-4324, I-84 Exit 376B.

PAYETTE, IDAHO

Lazy River RV Park, (208) 642-9667, four miles north on Highway 95.

RESTAURANTS

MONTPELIER, IDAHO

Butch Cassidy's, (208) 847-3501, 230 N. 4th St. Steaks, seafood and prime rib.

Ranch Hand Cafe, (208) 847-1180, two miles north on Highway 30. Hearty meals at rustic truck stop. Open 24 hours.

SODA SPRINGS, IDAHO

Betty's Cafe, (208) 547-4802, west of town cn Highway 30.

Brass Lantern Pizza Parlor, (208) 547-4575, Mountain View Mall. Pizza, burgers, chicken, seafood.

Ender's Cafe & Hotel, (208) 547-4980, 76 S. Main. Salad bar, daily specials.

LAVA HOT SPRINGS, IDAHO

Chuckwagon Restaurant, (208) 776-5626, 211 E. Main. Seafood, homemade pies.

Lazy A Ranch, (208) 776-5035, west on Highway 30. Chuckwagon dinners with campfire songs Monday through Saturday.

Royal Hotel, (208) 776-5216, 11 E. Main. Specialty is pizza.

POCATELLO, IDAHO

Buddy's, (208) 233-1172, 626 E. Lewis, Idaho State University favorite serves pizza, pasta.

Cowboy Cafe, (208) 232-1966, 3256 Highway 30. Hearty food, open 24 hours weekends.

Elmer's Pancake & Steak House, (208) 232-9114, 851 S. 5th St. Family dining with homemade food.

Frontier Pies, (208) 237-7159, 1205 Yellowstone Ave. Popular regional chain restaurant.

Grecian Key, (208) 234-0015, 314 N. Main. Greek food prepared tableside.

Mama Inez, (208) 234-7674, 450 Yellowstone Ave. Authentic Tex-Mex food.

Remo's, (208) 233-1710, 160 W. Cedar. Fresh pasta and seafood, steaks, extensive wine list, outdoor dining in summer.

The Sandpiper, (208) 233-1000, 1400 Bench Road. Prime rib, steaks, seafood.

AMERICAN FALLS, IDAHO

Lakeview Cafe, (208) 226-2194, Interstate 15.

Melody Lanes Bowl Cafe, (208) 226-2815, 152 Harrison. Local favorite for lunch.

Mr. G's Golden Fried Chicken, (208) 226-5951, 616 Fort Hall Ave.

Waterfront Restaurant, 2730 Marina Road. Steaks and seafood.

RUPERT, IDAHO

The Wayside, (208) 436-4800, Highway 24 and I-84

BURLEY, IDAHO

China First Restaurant, (208) 678-9399, 901 Overland. Chinese, American and Vietnamese food.

Connor's Cafe, (208) 678-9367, I-84 Exit 208. Fresh baked goods. Open 24 hours.

Price's Cafe, (208) 678-5149, 2444 Overland Ave. Home-cooking, smorgasbord.

Tio Joe's, (208) 678-9844, 262 Overland Ave. Tex-Mex.

HANSEN, IDAHO

South Hills Saloon & Restaurant, (208) 423-6339, Highway 30.

KIMBERLY, IDAHO

Maxie's Pizza and Pasta, (208) 423-5880, 626 Main N.

TWIN FALLS, IDAHO

Aroma, (208) 733-0167, 147 Shoshone St. N. Italian cuisine, seafood.

The Buffalo Cafe, (208) 734-0271, 218 4th Ave. W. Locally popular for breakfast and lunch.

Depot Grill, (208) 733-0710, 545 Shoshone St. S. Lunchtime smorgasbord. Open 24 hours.

La Casita, (208) 734-7974, 111 South Park Ave. Mexican food, fast service.

Peking Restaurant, (208) 733-4813, 824 Blue Lakes Blvd. N. Variety of Chinese specialties.

Rock Creek, (208) 734-4154, 200 Addison Ave. W. Steaks, seafood, salad bar. Fine dining in informal setting.

Sizzler, (208) 733-8650, 705 Blue Lakes Blvd. N.

BUHL, IDAHO

Home Plate Cafe, (208) 543-4187, 114 Broadway Ave. S.

Ramona Restaurant, (208) 543-8440, 113 Broadway Ave. S. Family restaurant located in former theater.

HAGERMAN, IDAHO

Frog's Lilypad, (208) 837-6227, State and Hagerman.

River Bank Restaurant, (208) 837-6462, 191 N. State. Specializes in catfish, salmon, and trout.

BLISS, IDAHO

Oxbow Cafe, (208) 352-4250, Highway 30.

GLENNS FERRY, IDAHO

Hanson's Cafe, (208) 366-9983, 201 E 1st Ave.

MOUNTAIN HOME, IDAHO

Carlos' Mexican Restaurant, (208) 587-2966, 1525 American Legion Blvd. Casual family dining.

Footnote Restaurant & Lounge, (208) 587-9796, 1130 Highway 20. Steaks and seafood.

The Gear Jammer, (208) 587-4465. I-84 Exit 95. Big truck stop, deli, bakery.

MOUNTAIN HOME, IDAHO (CONT.)

Stoney's Desert Inn, (208) 587-9931, two miles east of I-84 at Exit 90. Favorite with locals and truckers. Open 24 hours.

BOISE, IDAHO

Amore, (208) 343-6435, 921 W. Jefferson. Creative Italian cuisine.

Brick Oven Beanery, (208) 342-3456, Fifth and Main. Lunch and dinner.

The Capri, (208) 342-1442, 2520 Fairview. Locally popular for breakfast and lunch.

Heartbreak Cafe, (208) 345-5544, 607 Main. Fresh seafood, gourmet salads, burgers.

Louie's, (208) 344-5200. An Idaho favorite, specializing in pizza and Italian food.

Onati-The Basque Restaurant, (208) 343-6464, 3544 Chinden Blvd. Basque specialties served family-style.

Peg-Leg Annie's, (208) 375-3050, 3019 Cole Road. Wide menu, family dining.

Wok-In Noodle, (208) 343-7262, 4912 Emerald and two other locations. Chinese food with carry-out available.

NAMPA, IDAHO

El Charro, (208) 467-5804, 1701 1st St. Inexpensive traditional Mexican food in out-of-the-way spot.

Golden Corral Family Steakhouse, (208) 466-1266, 623 Caldwell Blvd.

House of Kim, (208) 466-3237, 1226 1st St. Korean and Szechwan cuisine.

Key Largo, (208) 466-8181, in the Karcher Mall. Steaks, prime rib, seafood.

Noodles, (208) 466-4400, I-84 and Franklin Boulevard. Pizza and Italian specialties. Also in Boise.

Say You Say Me, (208) 466-2728, 820 Nampa-Caldwell Blvd. Big omeletes and sandwiches. Breakfast and lunch only.

CALDWELL, IDAHO

Asia Restaurant, (208) 459-4303, 703 Main. Chinese and Japanese cuisine.

Cattleman's Livestock Cafe, (208) 454-1785, 1900 E. Chicago. Here's the beef.

La Bamba Restaurant, (208) 454-0057, 320 N. Kimball. Mexican food.

Mancino's Pizza, (208) 459-7556, 2404 E. Cleveland Blvd.

PARMA, IDAHO

Big Ben's Golden Wheel Drive-In, (208) 722-5284, 203 N. 9th Ave. Ice cream, sandwiches, and such.

Fort Boise Inn and Cafe, (208) 722-6014, 303 Main.

Fort Boise Pizza Emporium, (208) 722-6048, 206 N. 1st.

J Bar K Drive-In, (208) 722-5463, 911 E. Grove Ave.

PAYETTE, IDAHO

Big C, (208) 642-4157, south of Payette. Features finger steaks and long hamburgers.

Keystone Pizza, (208) 642-9333, 17 S. 8th.

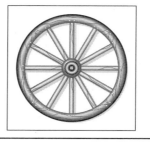

CHAPTER SEVEN

TRAIL'S END: OREGON

*"Friday, Oct. 27: Arrived at Oregon City at the falls of the
Willamette. Saturday, Oct. 28: Went to work."*
—Emigrant James Nesmith, 1843

FAREWELL BEND

When they crossed into what is now Oregon, the emigrants had
already traveled 1,510 miles and had more than four hundred miles—or
about another month on the road—left to go. Ahead of them lay the most
varied terrain of their trip: More stark desert, lofty mountains, cool forests, and raging rivers. Modern-day Oregon presents the same shifting
visual panorama, but while the pioneers viewed it as one last frustrating
stretch to their final destination, today's travelers can sit back, relax, and
enjoy the ride across this scenic state.

The first notable trail landmark inside Oregon is at **Keeney Pass**,
sometimes known as Lytle Pass. Here, one-half mile of deeply worn ruts
may be seen through the pass. The BLM has erected interpretive panels
at the site, which is six miles southeast of Vale.

The Malheur River runs south of Vale, and its name means "un-
lucky" in French. Indeed, this is where the travelers following Stephen
Meek left on their ill-fated trek across uncharted territory to avoid the
Blue Mountains. Nearby, another unfortunate, John D. Henderson, is

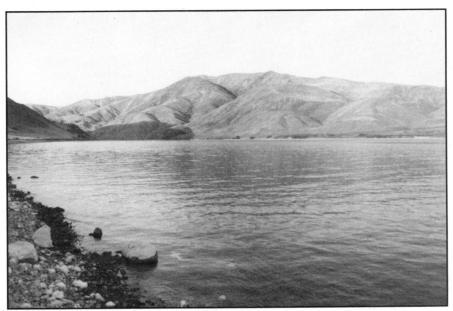

Farewell Bend is where emigrants left the Snake River to begin their trek across Oregon. Julie Fanselow photo.

buried below the gravel road which parallels Lytle Boulevard. The monument marking his grave says that he died of thirst in 1850, unaware he was within sight of the river. But local historians contend that is not true. Reportedly, the story was concocted by a very creative elementary school student in Vale. Today, the area's history is remembered each August with the Malheur County Oregon Trail Cultural Festival, a weekend's worth of events which include wagon train rut tours, games and contests, a barbecue, and entertainment.

After traveling some twenty-five miles across this dry, dusty land, the emigrants once again arrived at the Snake River. This would be their last view of the river they had followed for more than 330 miles, so the area became known as **Farewell Bend,** and it was an important landmark for the emigrants. Today, the site is occupied by a popular Oregon state park best reached via I-84. Those who travel U.S. Highway 20/26 from Parma to Vale should backtrack to Ontario and the interstate, then head west. The Oregon welcome center at the Ontario rest area offers the first of many excellent trail interpretive sites along I-84 in Oregon. Be aware that Ontario is on Mountain time, while the Pacific time zone starts about twenty miles west, just before Farewell Bend.

Farewell Bend is at Exit 353, and travelers get a great view of it from the highway. Interpretation at the park itself is somewhat limited, but there are good trail ruts nearby and the park does have good boating, fishing, and camping opportunities. The author will never forget a night spent here in the summer of 1992. About an hour after crawling into my tent for the night, I went out for a trip to the restroom and saw an incredible array of stars in the unpolluted desert sky. I hauled my sleeping bag out of the tent and happily fell asleep by counting—not sheep—but shooting stars.

"We descended to the Snake River—here a fine-looking stream with a large body of water and a fine current; although we hear the roar and see below us the commencement of rapids where it enters among the hills," John Fremont wrote on his visit in 1843. "It forms here a deep bay, with a low sand island in the midst; and its course among the mountains is agreeably exchanged for black volcanic rock." The rapids noted by Fremont have been swallowed up by the Hells Canyon Dam downriver.

Just across from Farewell Bend is a point called Olds Ferry, established at the time of the Idaho gold rush to link the Oregon and Idaho sides of the Snake River above Hells Canyon. Late Oregon Trail emigrants may have used the ferry after taking an extended detour on Goodale's Cutoff (which ended for most emigrants near Bonneville Point). The nearby sand dunes and badlands are somewhat reminiscent of those near Scottsbluff, Nebraska.

To view the Oregon Trail ruts, head north from Farewell Bend State Park toward the town of Huntington on U.S. Highway 30. The remnants appear intermittently on the left side of the road, along with a small iron cross that marks the site where several emigrants were possibly killed by Indians in 1860. The traveler can return to I-84 via Exit 345 at Huntington, an old railroad town. Most Huntington residents now work in the nearby lime quarry and cement plant.

Farewell Bend has one of a few state park campgrounds in Oregon open year-round. For more information on the park, call (503) 869-2365. From Huntington, it's a forty-mile drive to Baker City, home of the National Historic Oregon Trail Interpretive Center at Flagstaff Hill.

SIDETRIP: HELLS CANYON

At Hells Canyon, the Snake River has carved the deepest gorge in North America—7,993 feet. The great depth comes courtesy of the river's neighbor to the east: Idaho's Seven Devils Mountain Range. The Hells Canyon National Recreation Area straddles the canyon and includes parts of the Wallowa Whitman National Forest in Oregon and the Nez Perce and Payette national forests of Idaho.

Three power dams—Brownlee, Oxbow, and Hells Canyon—and their reservoirs lead downriver to the canyon. When Congress created the recreation area in 1975, it saved some of the best whitewater rapids in the

United States by protecting sixty-seven miles of the Snake River. Congress also set aside 215,000 acres as the Hells Canyon Wilderness, with an outstanding network of trails open only to hikers and horseback riders.

Abundant in fish, wildlife, and geologic splendor, Hells Canyon is a sight to see. Sturgeon up to twelve feet long swim the depths of the Snake River. Elk, mule deer, bighorn sheep, cougar, bobcat, bear, and smaller mammals patrol the mountainsides. More than thirty outfitters offer float, jet boat, or whitewater trips through the canyon. For a list, contact the Hells Canyon National Recreation Area headquarters in Clarkston, Washington, at (509) 758-0616. (The number for boat trip reservations is (509) 758-1957.) Private rafters and jet-boaters may also ply the area, but a Forest Service permit is required before launching.

Hells Canyon can be accessed via I-84 Exit 356 between Ontario and Huntington (which feeds into U.S. Highway 95 at Weiser, then Idaho Highway 71 at Cambridge); via Oregon Highway 86 (which takes off east from I-84 Exit 302 at Baker City); or by way of Oregon Highway 82 from La Grande to Joseph. From Joseph, it is possible to go to Hat Point, a 6,982-foot canyon overlook on Forest Service Road 4240 via Imnaha. This steep, narrow, and rough road is not recommended for trailers.

FLAGSTAFF HILL

After leaving Farewell Bend, the emigrants had to travel through **Burnt River Canyon**, which proved a significant obstacle. It often took wagon trains five or six days just to negotiate the climb out of the canyon. Although it wasn't as steep as some other areas along the trail, the twisting canyon crossed several ravines. Food was scarce for both humans and livestock, which further depleted everyone's strength. Emigrant James Nesmith called the canyon "the roughest country I ever saw."

Today, I-84 takes the same narrow path. The Weatherby rest area just past Farewell Bend offers interpretation of the area, along with a small stone shelter about seven feet high which bears a plaque commemorating "Rattlesnake Springs—Old Oregon Trail 1843-1857." The spring doesn't flow, but kids may have a good time pretending the shelter is a castle.

About six miles northwest of present-day Durkee, the trail leaves what is now the interstate and heads for the area known as Virtue Flat. To rejoin the trail, modern travelers must continue on I-84 to Baker City and take Exit 302 to Oregon Highway 86. From here, head five miles east to the BLM's National Oregon Trail Interpretive Center at **Flagstaff Hill**.

The interpretive center opened Memorial Day Weekend of 1992, and 90,000 people had toured the facility just two months later. It's easy to understand why: The center has something for everybody, from senior

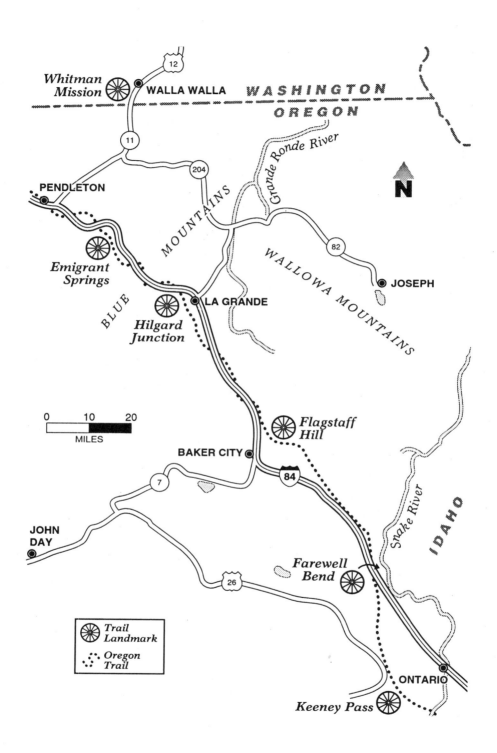

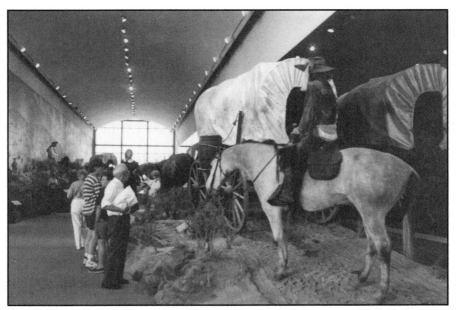

The National Historic Oregon Trail Interpretive Center has many exhibits that give insight into emigrant life along the trail. Julie Fanselow photo.

citizens who may remember their own grandparents' tales of trail travel, to youngsters who are asked to help "pack the wagon" for the trip west.

Upon entering the center, continue straight ahead. On both sides of a 100-foot walkway, dioramas offer a glimpse of what life was like on the Oregon Trail. Hired hands set the wagons a-rolling. A woman weeps at her baby's grave. Another young child teases a nanny goat and muses aloud "I wonder if I'll go to school in Oregon." Indians on a bluff warily survey the swelling emigration as it passes beneath them.

From large windows at the end of this display, visitors have a fifteen-mile view of the trail as it descended Flagstaff Hill and rolled toward the Blue Mountains, now plainly visible in the distance to the right. (The mountainous region straight ahead is Elkhorn Ridge.) The trail crossed this scene from the left through a draw and on over the alkali flat to the right.

From this viewpoint, the displays continue, each examining new aspects of the emigration as the wagons roll ever westward. Videos and exhibits show how the trains organized, how women and children fared along the way, how the travelers accomplished their most difficult river crossings, and what they did when they finally reached their destination. Beautiful photos and paintings of sites along the trail are interspersed with quotations from emigrant diaries. And near the end of the exhibits, visitors are invited to write a few words about how their own families made the trip west.

Other activities at the interpretive center include a network of hiking trails that lead down to the wagon ruts. The total distance is about two miles, depending on which route is taken, and hikers are encouraged to walk early in the day, if possible, when it's still fairly cool. (Summer daytime temperatures in eastern Oregon frequently surpass 90 or even 100 degrees.) Pioneer encampment and lode mine living history sites operate outside on a seasonal basis during the summer, and other special presentations are held on occasion in the indoor theater and outdoor amphitheater.

The interpretive center is open daily from 9 a.m. to 6 p.m. seven days a week. Admission is free, but donations are welcome (and deserved). For more information, call the center at (503) 523-1843.

One former trail landmark that is now long gone was the Lone Pine, which stood about five miles north of present-day Baker City on a branch of the Powder River. It was indeed the only tree for miles, and the earliest emigrant parties camped near it—until someone cut it down for firewood. Fremont, arriving in 1843, wrote that "on arriving at the river, we found a fine tall pine stretched on the ground, which had been felled by some inconsiderate emigrant ax. It had been a beacon on the road for many years past." In *The Oregon Trail Revisited*, Gregory Franzwa reported that the mayor of Baker City planted another tree at the site in 1945, but it did not survive.

Baker City got its start when gold was discovered in 1861 by miners who sere seeking the mythical Blue Bucket mine. The Armstrong nugget, weighing eighty ounces, was unearthed nearby and is now displayed at the U.S. National Bank. The gold rush was responsible for much of the ornate architecture in Baker City, which boasts more than 135 buildings on the National Register of Historic Places. Maps and brochures for self-guided walking or driving tours are available from the Baker County Visitor and Convention Bureau at 490 Campbell St. (Call (800) 523-1235 for information in advance.)

The Oregon Trail Regional Museum at Campbell and Grove streets has several notable exhibits, but none quite as fascinating as its collection of rocks, minerals, and semi-precious stones including many unusual "picture" cabochons. The Sumpter Valley Railroad, twenty-two miles west of Baker City on Oregon Highway 7, travels through the historic gold mining district and a wildlife sanctuary begun after dredging left the land ill-suited for farming. The powder-rich Anthony Lakes region thirty-five miles northwest of Baker City is a favorite with local snow skiers, but year-round use includes camping, fishing, and llama trekking.

It was between present-day Baker City and La Grande that Marie Dorian, a member of the Wilson Price Hunt party of Astorians, gave birth to her little boy in 1811. It hardly slowed her—or the party—down. Hunt, describing the event, wrote that Dorian "rode horseback with her newly born child in her arms. Another child, two years old and wrapped in a blanket, was fastened by her side. One would have thought, from her behavior, that nothing had happened to her."

La Grande, a forty-mile drive from Baker City, is another charming eastern Oregon town. Set in the spacious Grande Ronde Valley (locally called "the Valley of Peace"), La Grande looks northeast to the Wallowa Mountains and west to the Blue Mountains. Some emigrants, upon crossing through this valley, didn't care to go farther (and indeed some modern travelers, after a few seasons in rainy western Oregon, came back to live here instead). "Oh, if the Grande Ronde was west of the Cascade Mountains, how soon it would be taken up," emigrant Elizabeth Dixon Smith wrote in 1847. Elizabeth Wood, another traveler, called the area "one of Nature's beauty spots." La Grande's Birnie Park once served as an emigrant campground. It is located along Gekeler Lane and C Avenue on the south side of town. Nearby B Avenue follows the same path taken by the emigrants so long ago.

La Grande's annual events include an Oregon Trail Days celebration in mid-August that features such activities as an Oregon Trail Olympics, a buffalo barbecue, and flights over the valley. Call the La Grande-Union County Chamber of Commerce at (800) 848-9969 for more information or a self-guiding brochure to area Oregon Trail sites. La Grande is also home to Eastern Oregon State College and serves as gateway to the many recreational areas in the Blues and Wallowas. From here, the emigrants headed west into the Blue Mountains—and hoped they'd make it across before the snow fell.

SIDETRIP: THE WALLOWA MOUNTAINS

With their 10,000-foot peaks and rugged terrain, Oregon's Wallowa Mountains and Eagle Cap Wilderness have earned the nickname, "the Switzerland of America." The Nez Perce Indians once called these lands home; now they are beloved by vacationers, artists, and outdoors enthusiasts.

The Wallowas can be reached via Oregon Highway 82 out of La Grande. It's a sixty-two mile drive to Enterprise, the Wallowa County seat, and another six miles to Joseph (named for Chief Joseph, leader of the Nez Perce). Joseph is packed with art galleries and shops. Valley Bronze, a local foundry, serves sculptors worldwide. South of Joseph, forest-lined, four-mile-long Wallowa Lake State Park is one of Oregon's largest, busiest, and most beautiful. Services and activities offered include a marina and cabins, campgrounds, water sports, a go-cart track, horseback riding, llama treks, and hiking trails.

Campground reservations, still something of a rarity in the inland Northwest, are a must at Wallowa Lake during July and August. They must be made by writing the park at Box 323, Joseph, OR 97846 beginning the second Monday each January. Requests should be accompanied by an $11 deposit, which includes $8 toward the first night's camping fees and a $3 non-refundable reservation service charge. For more information or current fees, call the state campsite information center, open March through Labor Day Weekend at (503) 238-7488 or (800) 452-5687 within Oregon. This office will not accept reservations but can offer information on campsite availability. To visit the Wallowas and avoid all this rigamarole, try one of the many other campgrounds and backpacking opportunities throughout the 2.3 million acre Wallowa-Whitman National Forest and Eagle Cap Wilderness.

A tramway—one of the nation's steepest and longest—climbs to the 8,200-foot level on Mount Howard. From this vantage point, visitors can see the Eagle Cap Wilderness, the rim of Hells Canyon, and Idaho's Seven Devils Mountains. The tram runs 10 a.m. to 4 p.m. daily Mid-June through Labor Day, with a limited schedule available after Labor Day, weather permitting.

Joseph has many annual special events including a vintage car cruise in June, rodeo and jazz festival in July, and a "rattlesnake and bear feed" in August. The Wallowa County Museum in downtown Joseph has exhibits on the area's rich history. For more information, visit the Wallowa County Chamber of Commerce at 107 S.W. 1st St. in Enterprise, or call (503) 426-4622.

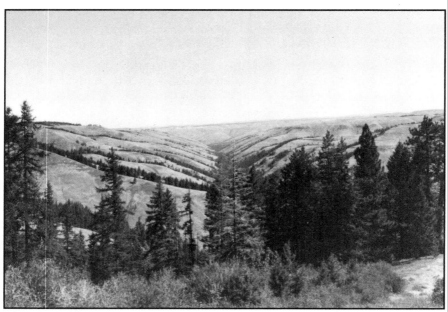

The view looking north from the Squaw Creek overlook in the Blue Mountains. Julie Fanselow photo.

THE BLUE MOUNTAINS

After heading west out of La Grande on I-84, the modern traveler quickly arrives at Hilgard Junction State Park on the Grande Ronde River. It takes about fifteen minutes to make the drive today; in the 1840s, emigrants often needed ten days to complete the same steep trip. Some historians (and a state interpretive panel at the park) say that this was probably an emigrant campground; others feel the Pioneer Springs 1.5 miles northwest was the more likely site. But it was from this general area that the pioneers began their ascent of the **Blue Mountains**.

Although it's possible to zip over the Blues from La Grande to Pendleton in about an hour, this beautiful, heavily forested area has a way of holding visitors captive. The emigrants were enthralled, too, by the tall conifer trees and the bracing air so unlike the desert heat they'd endured all summer. "Indeed, I do not know as I was ever so much affected by any scenery in my life," Narcissa Whitman wrote in 1836, comparing the area to her Eastern home. "The singing of birds, the echo of voices of my fellow travelers as they went scattered through the woods, all had a strong resemblance to bygone days." True, the terrain meant a long, tough climb. But firewood was no longer scarce, and the abundance of game, berries, and other edible wild plants meant delicious additions to the emigrants' meals.

Most travelers arrived at the Blues in late August or early September, before the heavy snows. Others weren't so fortunate. "While in the valley (the Grande Ronde), the snow fell to the depth of three feet, and on the Blue Mountains it was five feet deep," wrote F.A. Chenoweth, who made the trip in 1849. "The road over the mountains...difficult in good weather, was now utterly impassible with wagons. Our only alternative was to leave wagons, teams, and other property, and make our way across on foot."

The Forest Service established a Blue Mountain Crossing Oregon Trail interpretive trail west of Hilgard Junction for the emigrant trail's 150th anniversary in 1993. To get there, take I-84 to Exit 248 and turn onto Oregon Highway 30 toward Kamela for a half-mile, then turn onto Forest Road 600. Follow the signs for the remaining 2.5 miles to the trailhead. There is a thirteen-foot clearance where FR 600 passes under the interstate.

The main Blue Mountain Trail is handicap-accessible and easy. Paved and just .5 mile long, it features interpretive panels with artwork and emigrant diary excerpts, as well as a good look at the Oregon Trail itself. Two spur loops can extend the hike a bit longer over more moderate terrain. Restrooms, drinking water, and a picnic area are available at the trailhead.

The small town of Meacham, at Exit 234, was named for emigrant Harvey Meacham, one of several pioneers buried in the area. In July

1923, President Warren Harding stopped here to commemorate the Oregon Trail's eightieth anniversary and drew a crowd of more than 12,000 people. A monument on the south edge of town memorializes all the unknown dead of the Oregon Trail.

Emigrant Springs State Park three miles northwest of Meacham marks the site where missionary Jason Lee discovered a good source of water in 1834. From that time on, the springs became a major campground for the travelers, and travelers can still camp there today. Five miles farther west, the trail wound straight through what is now the Deadman Pass rest area. Deadman Pass didn't get its name until the Bannock War several decades after the Oregon Trail heyday. A foot trail from the rest area leads to a short stretch of wagon ruts. Look for the sign near the westbound rest area exit (which is accessible via an interstate underpass from the eastbound rest area). A road from the eastbound area leads to a beautiful overlook of Squaw Creek Canyon.

After Deadman Pass, the emigrants left what is now I-84 to head down the mountain in a northwest direction. Many pioneer diarists mentioned the sweeping view of the Umatilla Valley and, in those days, Mount Hood, Mount Adams, and Mount Saint Helens. "The sight from this mountain top is one to be remembered," John Minto wrote in 1844. "It affects me as did my first sight of the ocean, or again, my first sight of the seemingly boundless treeless plains before we saw the Platte River." The valley view is still there, but modern dust and smog have unfortunately obscured the Cascade peaks.

The trail divided below, with one branch pressing westward across the Columbia Plateau and the other heading north to the Whitman Mission. Although a few obstacles remained, the emigrants had put one of their biggest worries—the Blue Mountains—behind them.

THE WHITMAN MISSION

In November 1834, the Rev. Samuel Parker traveled around New York State asking for missionaries to go west with him the following spring. In Wheeling, N.Y., Marcus Whitman—a country doctor for twelve years—agreed to make the trip. Together, they got as far as the Green River, where Whitman decided to return to the States to prepare for a trip the following year—a trip designed to establish the **Whitman Mission**.

The next spring, Whitman set off anew. With him were two things that would forever alter the course of American history: A wagon, which he was determined to take all the way west, and his bride, Narcissa Prentiss Whitman. She, too, had heard Parker's speech two autumns before and had long yearned to make the trip. Narcissa made it all the way, and with Eliza Spalding—another missionary's wife—was the first

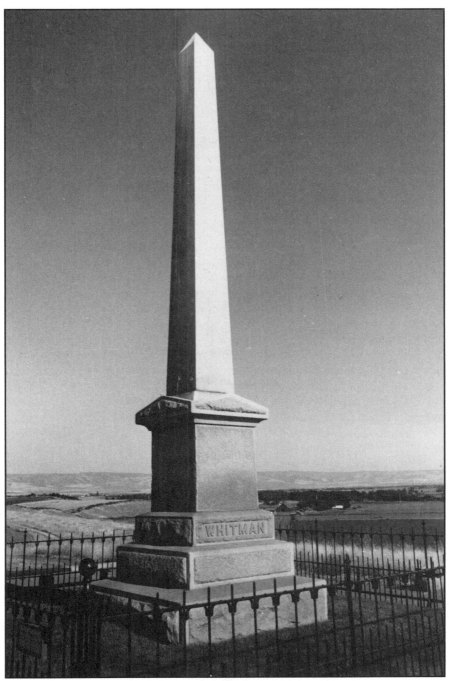

The monument of Whitman Mission commemorates the collision of the native people of the West and those who pursued religious zeal and America's "manifest destiny." Julie Fanselow photo.

white woman to cross the continent overland. The wagon was converted to a cart in Idaho and later traveled as far as Fort Boise, farther than any other wheeled vehicle before it. These successes inspired many frontier families to try the trip themselves.

Together, the Whitmans founded Waiilatpu, "Place of the Rye Grass," on the banks of the Walla Walla River. For the next decade, they would serve as missionaries, teachers, and friends to the Cayuse Indians. Their efforts brought only limited success and were destined to end in tragedy. In the meantime, however, the mission served as an important station on the Oregon Trail during the emigration's first few years. Travelers stopped for rest, supplies, medical treatment, and the Whitmans' hospitality. The mission was the birthplace of Alice Clarissa Whitman, born three months after the Whitmans' arrival. Sadly, the baby drowned in the Walla Walla just two years later.

Whitman thought that for his mission to succeed, he needed to change the Cayuse's nomadic ways. He encouraged them to farm, but few went along. The Cayuse were also indifferent to religious books, worship, and school. By 1842, reports of the mission's troubles caused Methodist officials back in the U.S. to order Waiilatpu closed. But Whitman, convinced the mission should stay open, made a midwinter ride back east to plea his case. Impressed by his commitment, the officials changed their minds.

Still, the cultural differences remained and—with the coming of ever more whites—deepened. In 1847, emigrants brought a measles epidemic that spread rapidly among the Cayuse, who had no resistance to the disease. Soon, half the tribe was dead. When Dr. Whitman's medicine helped whites but not Indians, many Cayuse believed they were being poisoned to make way for the pioneers. On Nov. 29, 1847, a band of Cayuse attacked the mission and killed the Whitmans and eleven others.

The Whitman Mission is an important stop along today's Oregon Trail since it shows, more than most sites, the collision between the native people of the West and those who pursued religious zeal and America's "manifest destiny." A small interpretive center tells the sad story from both sides. On one hand, the Whitmans were genuinely interested in the Cayuse and their welfare. On the other hand, they could not understand the centuries-old Cayuse practice of hunting and gathering on seasonal rounds. What seemed like aimless wandering to whites was the Cayuse's way of honoring the creator and the food they'd been provided.

Other sites at the Whitman Mission include a great grave in which the massacre victims were buried and an excavated area where early mission buildings are outlined. Visitors can get a good view of the entire grounds by taking the short, steep walk to the Whitman Memorial Shaft. From the top, you can see all of Waiilaptu, as well as the Blue Mountains, still stretching northward. Living history demonstrations featuring pioneer and Indian crafts are given on summer weekends.

Whitman Mission is open daily from 8 a.m. to 6 p.m. June through August and from 8 a.m. to 4:30 p.m. the rest of the year. Admission is $1 per person, with senior citizens and children under 16 admitted free. To find the site, take Oregon Highway 11 north from I-84 Exit 213 (just east of Pendleton). Walla Walla is forty-five miles north, and the mission is located seven miles west of town on U.S. Highway 12. Call (509) 522-6360 for more information.

From Whitman Mission, travelers can either return to Pendleton and parallel the Oregon Trail across the Columbia Plateau or save a little time by continuing west on Highway 12 to U.S. 730, which winds along the Columbia River to I-82 (which, in turn, connects with I-84 just a few miles south).

Walla Walla, meaning "many waters" or "small rapid stream," grew up in the wake of the Whitman Mission and is now a thriving city of 26,000. Its sights include the Fort Walla Walla Museum Complex with its exhibits on pioneer and agricultural life and Pioneer Park, which features duck ponds, an exotic bird display, a playground, swimming pool, and tennis courts. Although primarily an agricultural and regional retail and service center, Walla Walla and its neighbor, College Place, are home to three colleges: Whitman College and Walla Walla College (both four-year schools) and the two-year Walla Walla Community College.

Walla Walla has an abundance of lodging and restaurants, although camping in the area is somewhat limited. Annual events include the Walla Walla Balloon Stampede, ethnic heritage festivals, horse shows, and a mountain man rendezvous. For more information, contact the Walla Walla Area Chamber of Commerce at (800) 743-9562.

Pendleton, with 15,000 people, is the biggest city in eastern Oregon. At one time, it had thirty-two saloons and eighteen bordellos and was considered the entertainment capital of the Northwest. Today, Pendleton is best known for its woolen mills and the famous Pendleton Round-Up, a festival of rodeos, parades, and pageantry held the second week in September.

Pendleton Underground Tours, based at 37 S.W. Emigrant downtown, offers two different guided tours of underground tunnels and businesses built by Chinese immigrants in the late nineteenth century. Attractions include the Shamrock Cardroom, a laundry, meat market, and brothel. Reservations are required; call (503) 922-3232 for more information.

The Oregon Trail center at Flagstaff Hill is only the first of four major new interpretive centers that are planned across Oregon. Another expected to be built on the Umatilla Indian Reservation east of Pendleton will explain how the Oregon Trail affected the native people of the West. Other centers are planned for The Dalles and Oregon City.

The Pendleton Woolen Mills at 1307 S.E. Court Place also offers tours Monday through Friday. The Round-Up Hall of Fame on the Round-Up Grounds showcases Western and Indian memorabilia, photographs, and artifacts, as does the Umatilla County Historical Society Museum at 108 S.W. Frazer. For sleep or a meal, consider that Pendleton has the largest concentration of restaurants and motels within the next 125 miles. Call the Pendleton chamber at (800) 547-8911 or (800) 452-9403 in Oregon) for more information on area events and attractions.

THE COLUMBIA PLATEAU

West of Pendleton, the arid climate and wide open spaces are reminiscent of southern Idaho. Here, the Oregon Trail moves farther away from the modern interstate than it has in many miles. But one site that is fairly close to I-84 is the **Umatilla River Crossing** at Echo, accessible via Exit 193.

The U.S. government established the Umatilla Indian Agency in 1851 to oversee the Cayuse, Umatilla, and Walla Walla tribes. The agency was destroyed during the Yakima Indian wars of 1855. Later, the Oregon Mounted Volunteers established Fort Henrietta on the site, but it was abandoned after raids attributed to the Indians, and then burned to prevent Indian occupation. Further settlement in the area was delayed until the gold rush of 1858, when the federal government stationed more troops in the area.

Today's town of Echo has about 500 residents. The town took its name from the daughter of its co-founder, J.H. Koontz. A small park sits near where the emigrants forded the Umatilla River. It has an informative historical display and several campsites and is home to the Fort Henrietta Days celebration each September. Echo is remarkably well-attuned to its Oregon Trail History for such a small town, and City Hall can provide visitors with friendly advice and several informative brochures including a map of area trail sites and a flier detailing the emigrant route from Pendleton to Arlington.

After crossing the Umatilla, the pioneers camped in what is now known as Echo Meadows west of the present-day town, where several stretches of ruts still exist. Another twenty-five miles west, the emigrants arrived at **Well Springs**, another heavily used campground now on the U.S. Navy's Boardman Bombing Range. Well Springs offered one of the few reliable sources of water on the dry stretch across the plateau. A 7.5-mile segment of trail ruts in this area was to be marked by the Oregon-California Trail Association in time for the trail's sesquicentennial, but folks are still supposed to call the Navy at (503) 481-2565 before hiking on this land.

Other traces of the trail still exist through **Fourmile Canyon** southeast of Arlington; near **McDonald Ford,** where the emigrants crossed the John Day River; and at several other locations across the Columbia Plateau. But one of the very finest remnants is just west of the town of Biggs, right off I-84. Get off the interstate at Exit 104 and head west on

U.S. Highway 30. The ruts are well-marked on the road's south side, and they are definitely worth a stop and maybe a picture or two. It was here that the emigrants, who had been traversing the plateau to the south, got their first view of the Columbia River.

Stay on Highway 30 to reach the state's Deschutes River Recreation Area. The original crossing was flooded by the construction of The Dalles Dam, but in its day, it was a dangerous ford. Oregon Trail ruts may still be seen climbing the hill on the river's west side. An Oregon state park, the Deschutes River Recreation Area, is a favorite for fishing, picnicking, and camping, and the Deschutes itself ranks among the state's most popular whitewater rivers. (The Rogue and Umpqua, in southwest Oregon, are the others.)

Highway 30 dead ends seven miles from Biggs at Celilo, a sacred Indian fishing ground inundated by The Dalles dam. From here, it's a short drive to the town of The Dalles.

THE DALLES

Until 1846, **The Dalles** was—in a sense—the end of the Oregon Trail, or at least the overland portion of it. At the time, emigrants could continue their journey only by floating down the Columbia River. Dams

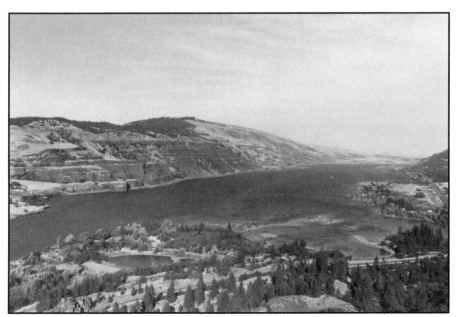

The rugged beauty of the Columbia River Gorge near the Dalles is still impressive today. Julie Fanselow photo.

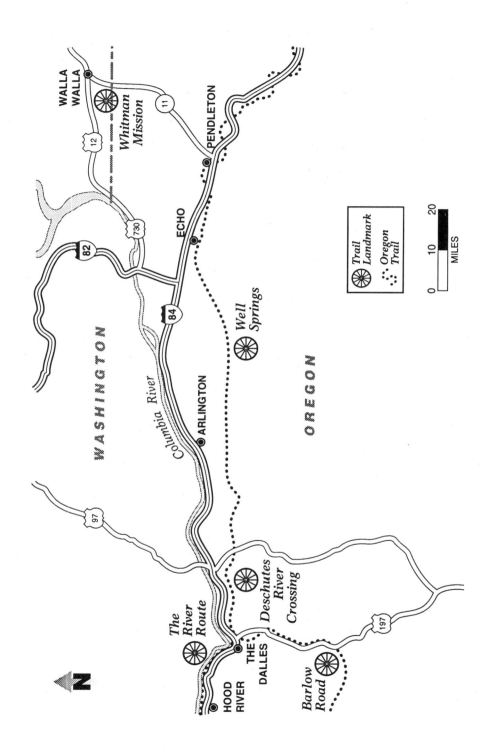

WALLA WALLA

Whitman Mission

11

PENDLETON

12

730

ECHO

82

84

Well Springs

WASHINGTON

Columbia River

ARLINGTON

OREGON

97

Deschutes River Crossing

The River Route

197

THE DALLES

HOOD RIVER

Barlow Road

N

Trail Landmark

Oregon Trail

0   10   20
MILES

have turned today's Columbia into one big series of reservoirs, but in the 19th century it was a river of treacherous rapids. Maneuvering rafts and livestock down the broad, swift river was quite difficult, to say the least. In fact, The Dalles got its unusual name from French trappers who called the area "les dalles," or "the trough" because of its once-wild character.

A park at 6th and Union streets in The Dalles bears a monument marking "The End of the Oregon Trail." Actually, emigrants choosing to brave the river would start their float at Chenoweth Creek, a protected harbor just west of The Dalles where rafts could be built and boats loaded.

The Dalles also was the site of an important Methodist mission started by Daniel Lee in 1838. This is where survivors of Stephen Meek's cutoff were taken and treated after their foolish trek in 1845. Until its closing in 1847, the mission also served other emigrants who stopped here to camp and resupply.

The Dalles Visitor and Convention Bureau at 901 E. 2nd St. (phone (800) 255-3385) has maps that detail self-guiding walking tours through the city's historic areas. A free train runs from town to The Dalles Dam, which offers daily tours in the summer. Other attractions include the Original Wasco County Courthouse at 406 W. 2nd St., which presents films on area history; the Wonder Works Children's Museum at 419 E. 2nd St.; and the Fort Dalles Museum, at 15th and Garrison streets in the last remaining building of a fort built in 1850 to protect emigrant traffic.

The Dalles is the gateway to the Columbia Gorge, recognized as an official national scenic area. This is a land of stunning waterfalls, varied recreational opportunities, fine restaurants, fun festivals, and roadside fruit stands. See the Columbia Gorge section for more information on things to see and do.

Beginning in 1846, the emigrants had to make a choice. They could take the river, or they could continue overland on the Barlow Road. Today's travelers face the same decision. Those in a hurry should probably opt for the river route, which parallels I-84. If time isn't a concern, consider the Barlow Road, which winds across the south shoulder of majestic Mount Hood. Either way is quite scenic!

SIDETRIP: CRATER LAKE NATIONAL PARK AND SOUTHWEST OREGON

Crater Lake National Park, about 250 miles south of The Dalles, is Oregon's only national park and one of its top scenic attractions. This once was the site of 12,000-foot Mount Mazama, a volcano, but eruptions about 6,850 years ago emptied the magma chamber beneath the mountain and caused the mountaintop to collapse, creating the depression which now cradles Crater Lake.

Crater Lake is America's deepest lake and one of its bluest. Its beauty is further enhanced by spectacular lava cliffs and forested slopes that rim the shore. Crater Lake is also a haven for wildlife. Bears, bald eagles, elk, mule deer, and more than 200 species of birds are among the species living in the national park.

The Rim Drive, a thirty-five-mile circuit around the lake, offers several wonderful views including those at the Sinnott Memorial (outside the visitor center) and Cloudcap. More than 100 miles of hiking trails are also available. A five-mile round-trip hike reaches Mount Scott, the parks' highest point at 8,926 feet, nearly 2,000 feet above the lake. A 1.1-mile trail leads to the boat landing at Cleetwood Cove, launching point for the Crater Lake Boat tours. These two-hour trips include information on Crater Lake's geologic and natural history; the prices are almost as steep as the Cleetwood trail at $10 for adults and $5.50 for those under age 12.

No license is required to fish at Crater Lake, and anglers might catch rainbow trout or kokanee salmon. Swimming is also permitted, but beware—the water is only fifty degrees! Crater Lake National Park has two first-come, first-served campgrounds with no hook-ups.

Bend, Oregon, is the largest town along U.S. Highway 97 en route to Crater Lake. Bend has been booming lately, thanks to its scenic setting near the Cascade Mountains and an influx of residents from the West's bigger cities. Just south of Bend, the High Desert Museum is one of the finest in the West, its indoor exhibits supplemented by more than twenty acres of outdoor trails. Visitors can see porcupine being hand-fed, stroll by an old settler's cabin, or learn about forestry.

Southwest of Crater Lake, the town of Ashland is home to one of America's premier theater companies, the Tony Award-winning Oregon Shakespeare Festival. Operating from mid-February through October, the festival annually performs eleven different plays ranging from Shakespeare's works to those of contemporary dramatists. Ashland is also known for its abundant art galleries, antique dealers, and boutique shopping.

For more information on these areas, contact Crater Lake National Park at (503) 594-2211; the Bend Visitors Center at (503) 382-3221; or the Ashland Chamber of Commerce at (503) 482-3486.

DOWN THE COLUMBIA

By the time they reached The Dalles, the emigrants were tired, broke, and more than ready to stop traveling. But they had one last hurdle to clear: the mighty **Columbia River**. Even after the Barlow Road was opened in 1846, late-arriving emigrants would sometimes find that way closed by snow. Then as before, the river remained the only option for getting to Oregon City.

People often spent days waiting to float down the Columbia. Some travelers built their own rafts of timber scattered near the river. Others opted to pay for a ride, but the price could be high—up to $50 or $100 per wagon, an exorbitant amount of money back then, particularly for emigrants who had been on the road for months. Livestock were often traded in lieu of cash payments.

At what is now the town of Cascade Locks, a prehistoric landslide had clogged the Columbia with piles of rocks, and most emigrants had to leave the river for a portage of three to five miles. Wagons that had been disassembled for the float were now rebuilt and repacked, then taken apart again once the cascades were past. Boats were typically floated right over the rapids and hauled ashore by Indians hired to help the process.

Samuel Parker, who emigrated to Oregon in 1845, wrote of arriving at the portage with an ill daughter. "I put my sick girl in a blanket and pack her and only rested once that day," he recalled. Larger craft such as steamboats could try to ply the rapids fully loaded, but it was a dangerous practice. Still, this was the last point of hardship for those who concluded their trip west via the Columbia River route. From here, all was smooth sailing. The Sternwheeler Columbia Gorge offers riverboat rides three times daily in summer, with departures at 10 a.m., 12:30 p.m., and 3 p.m. Take Exit 44 off of I-84 East. Call (503) 223-3928 for ticket prices and other information.

Many emigrants on the river route stopped at **Fort Vancouver**, established by the Hudson's Bay Company in 1824. This represented a bold move by the HBC, which hoped to secure Britain's claim to Oregon by moving its Northwest headquarters inland from the mouth of the Columbia. That may have been the case had the fort not been run by John McLoughlin, a kind-hearted Canadian who welcomed emigrants to Fort Vancouver and gave them supplies, often on credit.

By 1846, Britain's hopes of claiming Oregon were dashed when the territory was divided along the 49th parallel (our current boundary), not the Columbia River, as the British had hoped. Fort Vancouver was on American soil. McLoughlin retired and moved to Oregon City, became an American citizen, and continued his charitable ways. Today, he is revered as "the Father of Oregon."

Fort Vancouver is now a national historic site. The fort's stockade and several major buildings have been reconstructed on their original locations. Visitors are welcome from 9 a.m. to 5 p.m. daily Memorial Day through Labor Day and from 8 a.m. to 4 p.m. the rest of the year. Admission is $1 per person or $3 for a family. This is the site of a gala Fourth of July celebration often called one of the Northwest's best. For more information about Fort Vancouver, call (206) 696-7655.

Fort Vancouver sits near an area known as Officers' Row, a stately promenade of Victorian homes which once served as residences for the U.S. Army post established near the site in 1849. The houses are now occupied by shops and professional offices. Marshall House, at 1310 Officers' Row, was named for Gen. George C. Marshall, architect of the post-World War II recovery plan. A tour of the house includes a video on the history of Officers' Row and of Vancouver's role in the military since 1850. Horse-and-buggy rides are available in the area, too.

Vancouver, the oldest city in Washington State, has a population of about 47,000. It sits right across the river from Portland, offering its residents what may be the best of both worlds: Life in a large metropolitan area combined with Vancouver's lingering small-town feel and easy access to recreation. Because of these attributes, Vancouver has twice been named an "All-American City." Other historical sites include the Pearson Air Museum at 1105 E. 5th St.; the Clark County Historical Museum at 1511 Main St.; and Covington House, an 1846 log cabin that once served as a schoolhouse. It is located at 4201 Main St.

Southwest Washington is filled with other attractions including Vancouver Lake; Salishan Vineyards in La Center; Battleground Lake State Park; Paradise Point State Park; the Ridgefield National Wildlife Refuge; and Mount Saint Helens National Volcanic Monument. Get a shopping fix at the Vancouver Mall, with more than 115 shops, restaurants, and theaters, or attend August's Clark County Fair, one of the nation's ten largest. For more information on Vancouver, contact the Vancouver/Clark County Visitor and Convention Bureau at (206) 693-1313.

Travelers who didn't stop at Fort Vancouver floated on to the mouth of the Willamette and, from there, on to Oregon City. To reach Oregon City today, take I-84 west to I-205, the beltway which circles Portland. Head south on I-205. Oregon City is at Exits 8, 9, and 10.

SIDETRIP: THE COLUMBIA RIVER GORGE AND MOUNT HOOD

What's your pleasure? Hiking? Sailboarding? Dining? Scenic drives? The eighty-mile long Columbia River Gorge National Scenic Area has all these and a lot more, all within easy reach of I-84 (for fast-laners) and Washington Highway 14 (for those who like to dawdle).

Waterfalls may be the Gorge's most popular draw. A few cascades, including lovely Multnomah Falls, may be briefly glimpsed from the interstate. But to really appreciate the falls, drive on to Troutdale and get on the Columbia River Scenic Highway, which runs twenty-two miles east to Ainsworth State Park. The highway was begun in 1913 and passes by Bridal Veil, Horsetail, and Multnomah falls, among others. Many

Gorge waterfall areas offer hiking opportunities, including the popular Eagle Creek Trail to Punch Bowl Falls and the Larch Mountain hike at Multnomah Falls. Stop at Crown Point and its Vista House for a great view of the Gorge and information on the area's history.

Hood River, a town of about 5,000 people, is the sailboarding capital of the world, and it sometimes seems every other car in town is piled high with sailboards, mountain bikes, kayaks, and other recreational gear. This is also big bungee jumping territory, and a local group called the Dangerous Sports Club is always on the lookout for new ways to risk life and limb. But Hood River has another side, too: It is home to an astounding array of great restaurants, ranging from the elegant (and expensive) Columbia River Court Dining Room in the Columbia Gorge Hotel to the Whitecap Brewpub, home of Full Sail Ales, traditional and unusual bar food, and live entertainment.

Hood River is also a jumping-off spot for Mount Hood, highest point in Oregon at 11,235 feet. The 1.1 million-acre Mount Hood National Forest offers more than 100 campgrounds and more than a thousand miles of hiking trails. Timberline, one of three ski areas at Mount Hood, actually offers skiing well into summer at an elevation of 8,500 feet.

The Hood River Scenic Railroad transports passengers from Hood River to Odell (seventeen miles) or Parkdale (forty-four miles) on twice-daily excursions. The train, built in 1906, offers views of Oregon's famous fruit orchards, towering Mount Hood and Mount Adams, and the beautiful Hood River Valley. Kids ride free on their birthday with proof of age, and special-event trips include a Father's Day Surprise and Western train robberies. Reservations are recommended; call (503) 386-3556 for more information.

Washington State also borders the Gorge, and boasts several great attractions of its own. The Maryhill Museum of Art near the Biggs Junction includes work by the French sculptor Auguste Rodin and an extensive collection of Native American baskets and artifacts. The museum was named for Mary Hill, wife of lawyer Sam Hill, who also built the nearby replica of England's famous Stonehenge.

Bonneville Dam has visitor centers on both its Washington and Oregon sides. The Washington center features views of the dam's generators and turbines; the Oregon side shows the workings of the Bonneville Locks. Both sides have fish-viewing areas from which trout and salmon can be seen negotiating the dam's fish ladders.

Carson Hot Springs Resort at the tiny town of Carson, Washington, offers very reasonable lodging and inviting creature comforts, including 126-degree natural mineral baths, massages, RV hook-ups (tent campers are welcome, too), and a restaurant. Folks have been flocking here for more than a century, and the baths are supposed to be good for whatever ails you. Call (509) 427-8292.

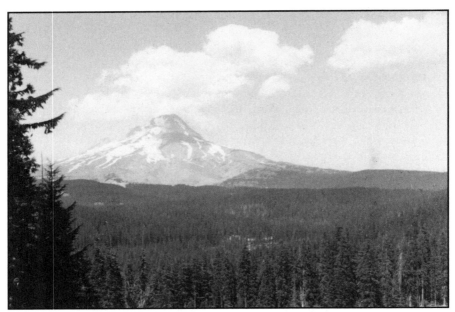

Views from the Barlow Road show 11,235-foot Mount Hood and its glaciers. Julie Fanselow photo.

For more information on the Columbia River Gorge, call The Dalles Convention & Visitors Bureau at (800) 255-3385 or the Hood River County Chamber of Commerce at (800) 366-3530. For information on Mount Hood, contact the Forest Service in Gresham at (503) 666-0700 or the Hood River Ranger District in Parkdale at (503) 352-6002.

THE BARLOW ROAD

Most early emigrants made it successfully down the Columbia River. But others lost their possessions, even their lives, in its raging rapids. Others were incensed by the high tolls charged by boatmen on the Columbia. Here they were, so close to the Willamette Valley and yet so far away. Could there be another route...a land passage around the great Mount Hood?

In 1845, two pioneer leaders—Samuel K. Barlow and Joel Palmer— decided to find out, and the result became known as the **Barlow Road**. Historians say Palmer intended to float down the Columbia until he heard the two ferry boats were engaged for at least ten days. He then learned Barlow had already set off to find a route 'round the mountain.

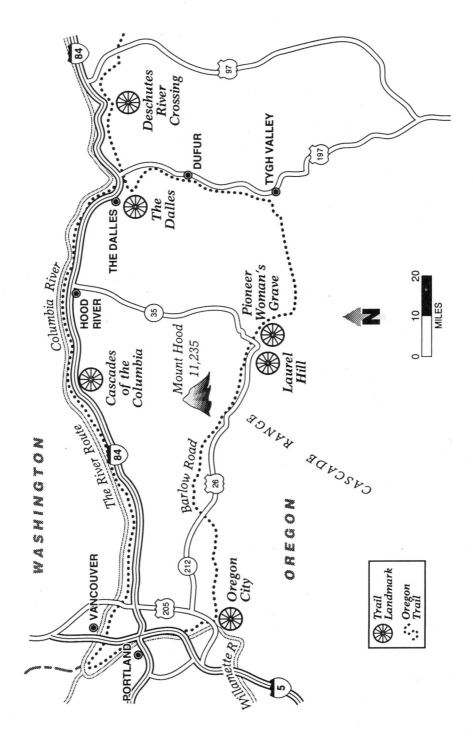

181

Palmer chased Barlow down, their parties camped together at Tygh Valley, then they set off to find the last link in the overland route.

It was tough going. Each day, members of the party would move out in advance to clear brush and timber, while Palmer, Barlow, and a few other men went still farther ahead to try and find the pass over the Cascades. It was October, and they were racing against time. The sun set earlier each evening, and the nights were bitterly cold. Food supplies dwindled, and the travelers were growing ever more weary.

By climbing Mount Hood, Palmer finally found the pass they were seeking, through Summit Meadows and the Zigzag River watershed. But snow was threatening, and the travelers decided to cache supplies at a place just east of the pass they called Fort Deposit and move on by pack team to the Willamette Valley.

Soon after reaching his destination, Barlow approached the Oregon provisional legislature, saying he would clear and maintain the road over the Cascades if officials would allow him to collect tolls. The deal was made, and the Barlow Road officially opened in time for the fall emigration season of 1846. That autumn, an estimated 145 wagons and nearly 1,000 wagons used the road that Barlow, Palmer, and their men had hacked out just the year before.

Barlow Road tolls amounted to five dollars per wagon and ten cents a head for livestock, much cheaper than passage down the Columbia River. But the trip was not for the faint of heart. "Toward noon, our roads became intolerable," Esther McMillan Hanna wrote in 1853. "I never could have imagined such roads nor could I describe it for it beggars description! Over roots and branches, fallen trees and logs, over streams, through sloughs and marshes, up hill and down—in short, everything that could possibly make it intolerable."

Today's traveler can view the Barlow Road much as it was in emigrant times. The Forest Service has done little to alter the route, meaning that it is as bumpy as Hanna described it. In the interest of time (and to preserve passengers' nerves and dental fillings), traverse only part of the Barlow Road.

To get there, take U.S. Highway 197 south from The Dalles to Tygh Valley, a distance of thirty-one miles. This is a beautiful road that roller-coasters up and down past fruit orchards and grain fields. At Tygh Valley, follow the signs to Wamic. Bear left into Wamic at the "Y" just before town. Follow the Barlow Road signs onto Forest Road 48. The road travels into, then out of, then back into Mount Hood National Forest. Finally, watch for a small brown sign indicating the Barlow Road, now known as Forest Road 3530.

Branded cedar posts mark the Barlow Road route today. The Forest Service planned to erect place name signs at several sites in time for the 1993 trail sesquicentennial. The agency also plans a new brochure featuring the road and a list of hiking opportunities in the area. For informa-

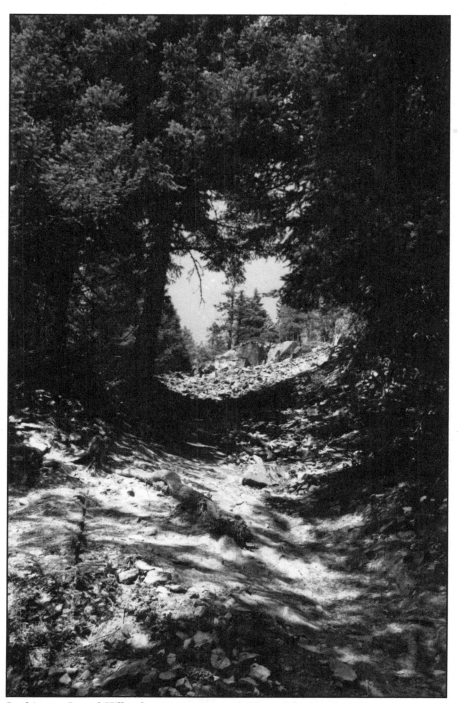

Looking up Laurel Hill today, it appears much like it did when the emigrants struggled up its grade. Julie Fanselow photo.

tion, write the Bear Springs Ranger District at Route 1, Box 222, Maupin, OR 97037.

Many emigrant parties camped east of the tollgate, and it became quite a dumping ground as the travelers sought to lighten their wagon loads before crossing the mountain. The next day, they'd press on as many as eighteen miles to the White River. This same stretch can be followed closely today, but at a pace of just ten to fifteen miles per hour. A few primitive campgrounds are scattered along the way.

Near White River Station, travelers can continue on the Barlow Road or cut over to Forest Road 48. The latter soon reaches Oregon Highway 35, the Mount Hood loop road from Hood River, which in turn soon merges with U.S. Highway 26. Forest Road 3531, two miles west of the White River East Snow Park on Highway 26, is the road to the **Pioneer Woman's Grave**, easily one of the most affecting sites along the Oregon Trail. The grave marks the burial site of a woman who died on the Barlow Road, and it has gradually developed into a mound of boulders and stones placed by passers-by. It's impossible to view this monument and not feel sorry for this unknown woman who came so close to her destination before finally succumbing to the trail's rigors. Barlow Pass and a good hiking segment of the old emigrant road are located near the grave, as is a trailhead for the Pacific Crest Trail.

Laurel Hill was loudly cursed by all who came upon it, and some travelers thought it was the most difficult passage of the entire trip. After returning to Highway 26 from Forest Road 3531, watch for a turn-out about six miles west on the left-hand side. This is the trailhead to Laurel Hill, which actually consisted of two chutes for a combined vertical drop of more than 300 feet and a grade of about sixty percent.

Standing at the bottom or the top of the scree-covered chute, it is hard to imagine how the travelers made it down this unbelievably steep slope. The round-trip hike up and back can easily be done in a half-hour today. Not so in the nineteenth century. Some emigrants took their vehicles apart and slid them down the grade. Others dragged felled trees behind the wagons as brakes. Still other travelers used long ropes, one end tied to the wagon, the other wound around a sturdy tree. They would then let out the rope ever so slowly, praying it would not break. For decades after trail travel ended, it was possible to see rope burns on several tree stumps along Laurel Hill, but the last of the stumps so marked reportedly rotted away in the 1970s.

A replica of the most recent Barlow Road tollgate (used from 1879 to 1915) stands about five miles west of Laurel Hill, along with a pleasant picnic grove and Forest Service campground built during the 1930s by the Civilian Conservation Corps. From here, the travelers rolled on west across the Sandy River. Many stopped for final rest and rations at the Phillip Foster Farm on Eagle Creek, now privately owned. Finally, they arrived at Oregon City, the end of the Oregon Trail.

SIDETRIP: PORTLAND ATTRACTIONS

With its views of the Cascades and plentiful parks, Portland is a city uncommonly blessed by nature. But Portland is more than just a pretty face. It is home to a progressive populace, an active arts scene, and loads of activities. Mix these with a keenly developed sense of humor: Long-time Mayor Bud Clark is possibly best known for the "Expose Yourself to Art" poster, which featured his honor in a trenchcoat flashing a statue.

Naturally, many Portland-area people spend their free time fleeing town to the slopes of Mount Hood or the beaches of the windswept Oregon Coast. But anyone deciding to stay and explore the city itself has plenty of options from which to choose. Portland is a city of parks, with 4,700-acre Forest Park on the west side leading the way. This beauty spot boasts hiking trails and picnic grounds with spectacular views of the city. It is also close to Washington Park, home of the acclaimed Oregon Museum of Science and Industry, the Metro Washington Park Zoo, the World Forestry Center, and an impressive Japanese Garden. Others seeking reflection may want to visit The Grotto, a religious sanctuary and botanical garden at N.E. 85th Avenue and Sandy Boulevard.

Weekends between March and December, the Portland Saturday Market beneath the Burnside Bridge offers wares from more than 250 artists, craftspeople, and fresh produce sellers. Food to eat on the premises and a wide array of entertainment are also available, and the market is open Sundays as well as Saturdays.

Portland's appreciation of history is reflected by the Oregon Historical Society museum at 1230 S.W. Park Avenue and by the James F. Bybee House, built in 1858 and restored to reflect life in Oregon in those heady post-trail days. It is in Howell Park on Sauvie Island, a rural refuge just north of Portland. Other museums include the Oregon Art Institute at 1219 S.W. Park Avenue, the Children's Museum at 3037 S.W. 2nd Avenue, the American Advertising Museum at 9 N.W. 2nd Ave., and the Oregon Maritime Center and Museum at 113 S. W. Front St.

Portland's arts and entertainment scene is really tough to beat. A constant stream of live popular musical acts parades through such venues as the Melody Ballroom, Roseland Theater, Key Largo, and innumerable small clubs. Chamber Music Northwest plays several times weekly during the summer on the Reed College campus, and outdoor jazz festivals abound during the warm months. Summer theaters present light and serious fare, and movie houses including the Northwest Film and Video Center and the KOIN Center downtown offer independent and classic film fare.

Special events in Portland include the Rose Festival, which takes place annually each June and lasts several weeks. Activities include parades, an air show, a hot air balloon festival, and much more. Downtown Portland is known for its public gathering places and eclectic architecture: Don't miss Pioneer Courthouse Square or Michael Graves' pastel Portland Building. The heart of the city also has a wealth of unusual shopping (or browsing) opportunities including Powell's Books, which takes up an entire city block, and Nike Town, an unabashed monument to the famous shoe manufacturer based in nearby Beaverton. What's more, Oregon has no sales tax, which means shopping in the Beaver State will saves several pennies on each dollar.

For more information on Portland-area attractions, call the Portland/ Oregon Visitors Association at (800) 345-3214 (or (503) 222-2223 inside Oregon). The state also maintains an "Oregon Welcome Center" at Exit 308 off of I-5 near the Oregon-Washington border.

OREGON CITY

By all rights, **Oregon City** should probably be called McLoughlin after John McLoughlin, the man who did more than any other to ensure the success of this town and, indeed, all of Oregon. From his base at Fort Vancouver, McLoughlin directed the building of several cabins at the falls of the Willamette River in the late 1820s. They were soon burned by Indians, but McLoughlin responded by building a sawmill and flour mill in 1832. Settlers continued to trickle in over the next decade, and in 1843

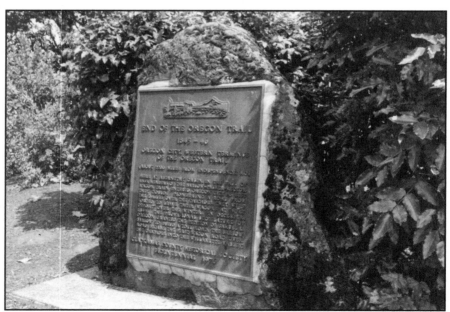

A trail-side plaque marks the end of the trail in Oregon City. Julie Fanselow photo.

they named Oregon City—which McLoughlin had named—the seat of their new provisional government.

Today, Oregon City is a suburb of the much-larger Portland, but it retains its claim to historical fame. Start a visit with a tour of the restored **McLoughlin House** at 713 Center St., where McLoughlin and his wife, Marguerite, lived after his retirement. They continued the tradition of hospitality they'd started at Fort Vancouver, opening their home to newly arrived emigrants, the needy, and the sick. The home is filled with beautiful period furniture, and the tour guides tell entertaining tales of McLoughlin's fascinating life. The house is open for tours from 10 a.m. to 4 p.m. Tuesday through Saturday and 1 to 4 p.m. Sunday except during the month of January, when it is closed. Admission is $2.50 for adults, $2 for seniors, and $1 for students ages six through seventeen. Call (503) 656-5146 for more information.

The **End of the Oregon Trail Interpretive Center** at Fifth and Washington streets is another fine, small museum tracing the trail's history and its impact on the young nation. A few exhibits here offer insight into aspects of the trail rarely covered elsewhere, such as clothing: Each emigrant had only two to three different outfits for the long trip. The museum is open from 10 a.m. to 4 p.m. Tuesday through Saturday and noon to 4 p.m. Sunday. (It, too, is closed during January.) Admission is $2 for adults, $1.50 for seniors, and $1 for ages six through seventeen. (Phone (503) 657-9336 for more information.) This facility will eventually be incorporated into a bigger interpretive center planned for Abernethy Green, which is where many emigrants—too poor to afford a room—camped upon reaching Oregon City. See the green and the end-of-the-trail monuments at the corner of Abernethy and Washington streets.

Each July, an outdoor Oregon Trail pageant is presented on the campus of Clackamas Community College. Titled "Oregon Fever," the show traces the adventures of several families who traveled together along the trail in 1851. Each performance is preceded by live musical entertainment, and several special events such as salmon bakes and pioneer history talks are scheduled each year. For more information, performance times, and ticket prices, call the Oregon City Chamber of Commerce at (800) 424-3002 or the pageant box office at (503) 657-0988.

By the mid-1840s, Oregon City was a thriving little town with all the comforts the emigrants had known back in "the States." And although the travelers had spent five to six months on the road by the time they reached Oregon City, few took much time to rest upon getting here. Most newcomers spent the winter at Oregon City, then fanned out come springtime across the Willamette Valley and beyond.

Americans have always been a restless breed, ever ready to move for fresh land, opportunity, or the mere thrill of going somewhere new. But here in Oregon, the restless young republic had moved as far west as it could go. Now the emigrants faced the challenges of staying put and of building new lives for themselves.

Industrious James Nesmith, quoted at the beginning of this chapter, became Oregon's first senator. Rachel Fisher Mills experienced the deaths of her husband and the youngest of their four children en route to Oregon, but here she remarried and had a second family. And Ezra Meeker, who traveled west as a young man in 1852, later retraced his route eastward, marking the way with monuments and asking all he met to remember and preserve the Oregon Trail and the brave emigrants who made the greatest peacetime migration in human history. It is unlikely this nation will ever forget.

LODGING

ONTARIO, OREGON

Holiday Motor Inn, (503) 889-9188, 615 E. Idaho Ave., $28-$30.

Motel 6, (503) 889-6617, I-84 Exit 376 or 376B, $36.

Ontario Best Western Inn, (800) 528-1234, 251 Goodfellow St., $47-$60.

Tapadera Motor Inn, (503) 889-8621, 1249 Tapadera Ave., $34-$40.

HUNTINGTON, OREGON

Farewell Bend Motor Inn, (503) 869-2211, I-84 Exit 353, $38.

BAKER CITY, OREGON

Best Western Sunridge Inn, (800) 233-2368, Sunridge Lane, $52-$62.

Eldorado Inn, (503) 523-6494, 695 Campbell St., $28-$39.

Green Gables Motel, (503) 523-5588, 2533 10th St., $23.

Oregon Trail Motel, (800) 628-3982, 211 Bridge St., $30-$34.

Royal Motor Inn, (503) 523-6324, 2205 Broadway, $31-$35.

Super 8, (800) 843-1991, 250 Campbell St., $34-$76.

LA GRANDE, OREGON

Broken Arrow Lodge, (503) 963-7116, 2215 E. Adams Ave., $28-$32.

Pitcher Inn Bed & Breakfast, (503) 963-9152, 608 N Ave., $55-$75.

Pony Soldier Motor Inn, (503) 963-7195, 2612 Island Ave., $55-$65.

Stange Manor Bed & Breakfast, (503) 963-2400, 1612 Walnut St., $45-$65.

Stardust Lodge, (503) 963-4166, 402 Adams Ave., $24-$30.

MILTON-FREEWATER, OREGON

Birch Tree Manor Bed & Breakfast, (503) 938-6455, 615 S. Main St., $45.

Jensen's Motel, (503) 938-5547, 104 N. Columbia (Oregon Highway 11), $30-$39.

WALLA WALLA, WASHINGTON

Comfort Inn, (800) 4CHOICE, 520 N. 2nd Ave., $55-$60.
Econo Lodge, (800) 446-6900, 305 N. 2nd Ave., $34.
Green Gables Inn Bed & Breakfast, (509) 525-5501, 922 Bonsella, $65-$90.
Nendel's Whitman Inn, (509) 525-2200, 107 N. 2nd Ave., $49.
Walla Walla Travelodge, (800) 255-3050, 421 E. Main, $48.

PENDLETON, OREGON

Best Western Pendleton Inn, (800) 528-1234, 400 S.E. Nye Ave., $46-$59.
Chaparral Motel, (503) 276-8654, 620 S.W. Tutuilla, $37-$43.
Let 'Er Buck Motel, (503) 276-3293, 205 S.E. Dorian, $19-$35.
Longhorn Motel, (503) 276-7531, 411 S.W. Dorian, $28.
Red Lion Inn, (800) 547-8010, 304 S.E. Nye Ave., $78-$88.
7 Inn, (503) 276-4711, I-84 Exit 202, $25-$40.

UMATILLA, OREGON

Heather Inn, (503) 922-4871, 705 Willamette Ave., $42-$55.
Tillicum Motor Inn, (503) 922-3236, 1481 6th St., $33-$39.

HERMISTON, OREGON

Posada Inn, (503) 567-7777, 655 N. 1st. St.
Sands Motel, (503) 567-5516, 835 N. 1st, $32-$38.
The Way Inn, (503) 567-5561, 635 S. Highway 395, $28-$32.

BOARDMAN, OREGON

Dodge City Inn, (503) 481-2451, 1st and Front streets, $35-$37.
Nugget Inn, (800) 336-4485, 105 Front St. S.W., $40.
Riverview Motel, (503) 481-2775, 200 Front St. N.E., $30-$38.

ARLINGTON, OREGON

Village Inn Motel, (503) 454-2646, Cottonwood and Beech streets, $35-$42.

BIGGS, OREGON

Best Western Riviera Motel, (800) 528-1234, West Main Street, $52-$62.
Biggs Nu Vu Motel, (503) 739-2525, I-84 and Highway 97, $29-$33.
Dinty's Motor Inn, (503) 739-2596, I-84 and Highway 97, $35.

THE DALLES, OREGON

Captain Gray's Guest House, (503) 298-8222, 210 W. 4th St., $45-$60.
Oregon Motor Hotel, (503) 296-9111, 200 W. 2nd St., $38-$40.
Shamrock Motel, (503) 296-5464, 118 W. 4th St., $28-$35.
Shilo Inn, (800) 222-2244, 3223 Frontage Road, $49-$90.
The Inn at The Dalles, (503) 296-1167, 3550 S.E. Frontage Road, $39-$42.
Williams House Inn, (503) 296-2889, 608 W. 6th St., $55-$75.

HOOD RIVER, OREGON

Best Western Hood River Inn, (800) 828-7873, 1108 E. Marina Way, $56-$83.

Hood River Hotel, (503) 386-1900, 102 Oak St., $59-$125.

Lakecliff Estate Bed & Breakfast, (503) 386-7000, 3820 Westcliff Drive, $75.

Love's Riverview Lodge, (503) 386-8719, 1505 Oak St., $39-$59.

Meredith Gorge Motel, (503) 386-1515, 4300 Westcliff Drive, $37-$42.

Prater's Motel, (503) 386-3566, 1306 Oak St., $29-$35.

Vagabond Lodge, (503) 386-2992, 4070 Westcliff Drive, $39-$58.

CASCADE LOCKS, OREGON

Bridge of the Gods Motel, (503) 374-8628, U.S. Highway 30, $30-$36.

Cascade Motel, (503) 374-8750, 300 Forest Lane, $37-$45.

Inn at the Locks, (503) 374-8222, 1280 Forest Lane, $45-$75.

Scandian Motor Lodge, (503) 374-8417, $34-$48.

TROUTDALE, OREGON

Motel 6, (503) 665-2254, I-84 Exit 17, $37.

Phoenix Inn, (503) 669-6500, 477 N.W. Phoenix Drive, $40-$55.

VANCOUVER, WASHINGTON

Best Western Ferryman's Inn, (800) 528-1234, 7901 N.E. 6th Ave., $52.

Mark 205 Motor Inn, (800) 426-5110, 221 N.E. Chkalov Drive, $50-$85.

Neridel's Suites, (800) 547-0106, 7001 N.E. Highway 99, $43-$48.

Vancouver Lodge, (206) 693-3668, 601 Broadway, $38-$42.

GREATER PORTLAND, OREGON

Best Western Sunnyside Inn, (800) 528-1234, I-205 Exit 14 (Clackamas), $60-$64.

Chestnut Tree Inn, (503) 255-4444, 9699 S.E. Stark (I-205 Exit 21A), $40.

Cypress Inn-Portland South, (503) 655-0062, I-205 Exit 12 (Clackamas), $62-$67.

Days Inn, (800)325-2525, I-205 Exit 14 (Clackamas), $54-$64.

Imperial Motel, (800) 452-2323, S.W. Broadway and Stark streets, $55-$70.

Red Lion Inn/Coliseum, (800) 547-8010, 1225 N. Thunderbird Way, $73-$80.

Shilo Inn/Lloyd Center, (800) 222-2244, 1506 N.E. 2nd Ave., $50-$59.

Sweetbrier Inn, (800) 551-9167, 7125 S.W. Nyberg (Tualatin), $57-$71.

MOUNT HOOD, OREGON

Huckleberry Inn, (503) 272-3325, Government Camp Business Loop, $45-$96.

Mount Hood Val-U Inn, (800) 443-7777, 87450 E. Government Camp Road, $59-$125.

Timberline Lodge, (800) 547-1406, six miles north of Government Camp, $52-$140.

OREGON CITY, OREGON

Inn of the Oregon Trail Bed & Breakfast, (503) 656-2089, 416 S. McLoughlin Blvd., $48-$78.

Jagger House Bed & Breakfast, (503) 657-7820, 512 6th St., $55-$60.

Lewis Motel, (503) 656-7052, 18710 S. Highway 99E, $23-$43.

Poolside Inn, (503) 656-1955, 19240 S.E. McLoughlin Blvd., $35-$65.

Val-U Inn Motel, (800) 443-7777, 1900 Clackamette Drive, $51-$61.

CAMPING

HUNTINGTON, OREGON

Farwell Bend State Park, (503) 869-2365, I-84 Exit 353.

BAKER CITY, OREGON

Lariat Motel & RV Center, (503) 523-6381, 880 Elm.

Mountain View Holiday Trav-L-Park, (503) 523-4824, 2845 Hughes Lane.

LA GRANDE, OREGON

Hilgard Junction State Park, nine miles west on I-84.

Hot Lakes RV Resort, (503) 963-5253, 65182 Hot Lake Lane.

Stonewood RV Park, (503) 963-8121, 1809 26th St. #41.

MEACHAM, OREGON

Emigrant Springs State Park, (503) 983-2277, I-84 Exit 234.

WALLA WALLA, WASHINGTON

Fort Walla Walla Campground, (509) 527-3770, west on Dalles Military Road.

PENDLETON, OREGON

Brooke RV Court, (503) 276-5353, 5 N.E. 8th St.

Stotlar RV Park, (503) 276-0734, 15 S.E. 11th St.

ECHO, OREGON

Fort Henrietta RV Park, (503) 376-8411, 10 W. Main St.

UMATILLA, OREGON

Hat Rock Campground, (503) 567-5719, east on U.S. Route 730 across from Hat Rock State Park.

BOARDMAN, OREGON

Boardman Campground & Marina, (503) 481-7217, I-84 Exit 164.

BIGGS, OREGON

Maryhill State Park, (509) 773-5007, I-84 Exit 104, across the Columbia River in Washington.

Deschutes River State Recreation Area, (503) 739-2322, west on Highway 30. Primitive sites.

THE DALLES, OREGON

Horsethief Lake State Park, (509) 767-1159, I-84 Exit 87, across the Columbia River in Washington. Primitive sites.

Memaloose State Park, (503) 374-8811, along I-84 (westbound access only)

HOOD RIVER, OREGON

Toll Bridge Park, (503) 386-6323, seventeen miles south on Oregon Highway 35.

Tucker Park, (503) 386-4477, four miles south on Oregon Highway 281.

Viento State Park, (503) 374-8811, eight miles west along I-84.

HOOD RIVER, OREGON (CONT.)

Wind Ranch Camping & Lodging, (509) 493-2312, across the river east of Bingen, Washington. ""Run by sailboarders for sailboarders."

Numerous Forest Service campgrounds are located in the Mount Hood National Forest south of Hood River. Call (503) 352-6002 for information.

CASCADE LOCKS, OREGON

Bridge of the Gods RV Park, (503) 374-8628.

Cascade Locks KOA, (503) 374-8668, two miles east on Forest Lane. Kamping Kabins.

Marina Park, (503) 374-8619, on the Columbia River.

BONNEVILLE, OREGON

Ainsworth State Park, (503) 695-2261, eight miles west on I-84.

Eagle Creek, (503) 695-2276, eastbound access only off of I-84.

PORTLAND, OREGON

Jantzen Beach RV Park, (503) 289-8753, 1503 N. Hayden Island Drive.

Portland Fairview RV Park, (503) 661-6871, 21401 N.E. Sandy Blvd.

Reeder Beach RV Park, (503) 621-3970, 26048 N.W. Reeder Road (Sauvie Island).

Trailer Park of Portland, (503) 692-0225, 6645 S.W. Nyberg Road (Tualatin).

WAMIC, OREGON

Pine Hollow Lakeside Resort, (503) 544-2271, 34 N. Mariposa Drive.

MOUNT HOOD, OREGON

Mount Hood RV Village, (503) 622-4011, 65000 E. Highway 26 (Welches).

RESTAURANTS

VALE, OREGON

Pasta Shoppe, (503) 473-3124, 130 Smith St. N.

Starlite Cafe, (503) 473-2500, 152 Clark St. N.

ONTARIO, OREGON

Brewsky's Broiler, (503) 889-3700, Ontario Town Square mall. Casual dining with microbrews.

Casa Jaramillo, (503) 889-9258, 157 S.E. 2nd. Mexican food.

Cheyenne Social Club, (503) 889-3777, 111 S.W. 1st St., Steaks, seafood.

Kings Table, (503) 889-3898, 2281 S.W. 4th Ave. Buffet dining.

New Far East Restaurant, (503) 889-3602, 44 N.E. 3rd. Cantonese, Polynesian, and American cuisine.

HUNTINGTON, OREGON

Farewell Bend Restaurant & Lounge, (503) 869-2281, I-84 Exit 353.

BAKER CITY, OREGON

Baker Truck Corral, (503) 523-4318, I-84 Exit 304. Homestyle cooking, open 24 hours.

Brass Parrot, (503) 523-4266, Main and Chruch. Mexican food in historic downtown Baker City.

Haines Steak House, (503) 856-3639, ten miles north on U.S. Highway 30. Closed Tuesdays.

Oregon Trail Restaurant, (503) 523-5844, 211 Bridge St.

Sumpter Junction, (503) 523-9437, 2 Sunridge Lane. American and Mexican food.

LA GRANDE, OREGON

Blue Mountain/Flying J Travel Plaza, (503) 963-3432, I-84 Exit 265. Open 24 hours.

Centennial House, (503) 963-6089, 1606 6th St. Fine dining in a house listed on National Register of Historic Sites.

Herman's Tavern, (503) 963-9921, 210 Depot St. Soups and sandwiches.

Hobo's Great Hamburgers, (503) 963-2534, 2102 Adams Avenue. Sandwiches, salad bar, seafood.

Mamacita's, (503) 963-6223, 110 Depot St. Mexican food.

Nature's Pantry, (503) 963-7955, 1907 4th St. Vegetarian deli.

Tropidara, (503) 963-4402, 1106 Adams Avenue. Steaks, seafood, salad bar, and Sunday brunch.

WALLA WALLA, WASHINGTON

The Homestead Restaurant, (509) 522-0345, 1528 Isaacs. Seafood, beef, and pasta.

Jacobi's Cafe, (509) 525-2677, 416 N. 2nd St. Italian, American, and vegetarian food.

Modern Restaurant, (509) 525-8662, 2200 Melrose. Cantonese and American dishes.

Olive Branch, (509) 529-7054, 103 E. Main. American and international cuisine.

Red Apple, (509) 525-5113, 57 E. Main. Steak and seafood.

PENDLETON, OREGON

Big John's Hometown Pizza, (509) 276-0550, 225 S.W. 9th. Pizza, salad bar.

Cimmiyotti's, (503) 276-4314, 137 S. Main. Italian and American fare.

Circle's Barbecue, (503) 276-9637, 210 S.E. 5th. Steaks, prime rib, seafood.

The Hut, (503) 276-0756, 1400 S.W. Dorian. Steaks and seafood.

Lee's Cafe, (503) 276-5819, 5th and S.W. Emigrant. Chinese and American food.

Mike's Place, (503) 276-6920, 435 S.W. Dorian. Homestyle cooking.

ECHO, OREGON

Echo Hotel Restaurant & Lounge, (503) 376-8354, Main and N. Dupont streets.

H & P Cafe, (503) 376-8573, 231 Main.

STANFIELD, OREGON

Stanfield Cafe, (503) 449-1127, 170 N. Main.

UMATILLA, OREGON

Olde Country Brand Restaurant, (800) 447-7529. Pot roast and ribs.

Rockin Robins, (503) 922-5160, 1501 6th. Steak and seafood in 1950s atmosphere.

BOARDMAN, OREGON

C & D Drive-In and Bakery, (503) 481-4981, 103 N. Main.

Sunset West Pizza and Subs, (503) 481-2555, 210 S.W. Main. Ice cream.

BIGGS, OREGON

Dinty's Cafe, (503) 739-2416, Biggs Junction. Open 24 hours.

Jack's Fine Foods, (503) 739-2362, Biggs Junction. Steaks, daily specials.

THE DALLES, OREGON

Casa Del Rio, (503) 298-4661, 1240 W. 6th St. Mexican food.

Dave's Hometown Pizza, (503) 296-2281, 809 Chenowith St. Pizza, chicken, pasta, microbrews.

Dobre Deli, (503) 298-8239, 308 E. 4th St. Croissants, soups, salads, and sandwiches.

Marcella's Pizza, (503) 296-4567, 1455 W. 6th St. Authentic Italian pizza baked in brick ovens.

Portage Inn Restaurant, (503) 298-5502, Dalles bridge junction. Overlooks The Dalles Dam. Weekend brunch.

Tugboat Annie's, (503) 296-3774, 822 W. 2nd. Prime rib and seafood.

Washington Street Cafe, (503) 296-1217, 409 Washington. Country-style breakfasts.

HOOD RIVER, OREGON

Bette's Place, (503) 386-1880, 416 Oak St. Locally popular breakfast and lunch spot.

Columbia Gorge Hotel, (503) 386-5566, 4000 Westcliff Drive. Northwest cuisine, "famous farm breakfast." Reservations advised.

The Gorge Cafe, (503) 386-8700, Port Marina Park. River view dining in casual atmosphere.

Kampai, (503) 386-2230, 113 3rd St. Japanese fare.

Mesquitery, (503) 386-2002, 1219 12th St. Variety of cuisines grilled over 100 percent mesquite wood.

Purple Rocks Art Bar & Cafe, (503) 386-6061, 606 Oak St. Breakfast and lunch.

Santacroce's Famous Italian Cafe, (503) 354-2511, 4780 Highway 35. Traditional Italian food.

Whitecap Brewpub, (503) 386-2281, 506 Columbia. English-style pub with live entertainment.

CASCADE LOCKS, OREGON

Charburger Restaurant, (503) 374-8477, 714 S.W. Wa-Na-Pa. View of the Columbia River.

TROUTDALE, OREGON

Tad's Chicken 'n Dumplins, (503) 666-5337. On the Crown Point Highway with view of the Sandy River.

VANCOUVER, WASHINGTON

The Crossing, (206) 695-3374, 900 W. 7th St. Prime rib, steak, seafood, and chicken.

Old Country Buffet, (206) 256-9420, in Vancouver Plaza. Family dining.

Olive Garden, (206) 256-8174, at the Vancouver Mall. Italian food and more.

PORTLAND, OREGON

Atwater's Restaurant, (503) 275-3600, 111 S.W. 5th Avenue. Great views atop U.S. Bancorp Tower.

Escape from New York Pizza, (503) 226-4129, 913 S.W. Alder. Locally famous pizza by the slice or the pie.

Esparza's Tex-Mex Cafe, (503) 234-7909, 2725 S.E. Ankeny. Lunch and dinner. Closed Sundays and Mondays.

Hamburger Mary's, (503) 223-0900, 850 S.W. Park. Funky local favorite near theaters.

Kells, (503) 227-4057, 112 S.W. 2nd Ave. Irish pub and restaurant.

KOIN Center Grill, (503) 295-2820, 213 S.W. Clay. Northwest cuisine.

Macheesmo Mouse, (503) 228-3491, 715 S.W. Salmon and five other locations. Authentic Mexican food.

Monte Carlo, (503) 238-7627, S.E. 10th and Belmont. Italian cuisine.

Sayler's Old Country Kitchen, (503) 252-4171, Stark at S.E. 105th. Giant steaks, prime rib, seafood, chicken.

Shenanigan's on the Willamette, (503) 289-0966, 4575 N. Channel (Swan Island). Seafood, Sunday brunch. River view dining.

OREGON CITY, OREGON

Art's Cafe, (503) 656-2122, 201 S. 2nd. Locally popular family dining.

Edgewater Restaurant & Lounge, (503) 655-5155, 1900 Clackamette Drive. American cuisine with view of the Willamette River.

Elmer's, (503) 655-1837, 1837 Molalla Ave. Family dining.

The Friendship, (503) 657-4507, 1003 N. Main St. Chinese restaurant.

La Hacienda, (503) 656-2210, Oregon City Shopping Center (Highway 99E). Mexican food.

Oregon City Subbs, (503) 640-5047, 705 Main St. Big sandwiches.

Shari's Restaurant, (503) 657-9183, 1926 McLoughlin Blvd.

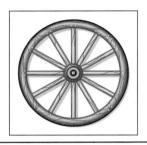

ABOUT THE AUTHOR

Julie Fanselow was born in Illinois and grew up in Bethel Park, Pennsylvania. She earned a bachelor's degree in journalism at Ohio University, where she minored in history and political science.

After 10 years as a reporter and editor for daily newspapers in Ohio, Washington state, and Idaho, Fanselow turned to full-time freelance writing in 1991. Her byline has appeared in numerous regional and national publications including: Entertainment Weekly, The Wall Street Journal, Nation's Business, Vegetarian Times, Outdoor Photographer, The (Cleveland) Plain Dealer, Seattle Weekly, Videomaker, Writer's Digest, Editor & Publisher and Ski. This is her first book.

Fanselow enjoys traveling, hiking, camping, reading, music and movies. She lives with her husband, Bruce Whiting, near the Oregon Trail in Twin Falls County, Idaho.

Out here–there's no one to ask directions

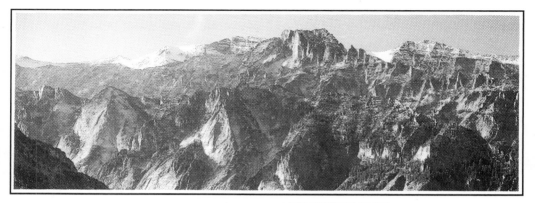

. . . except your **FALCON**GUIDE.

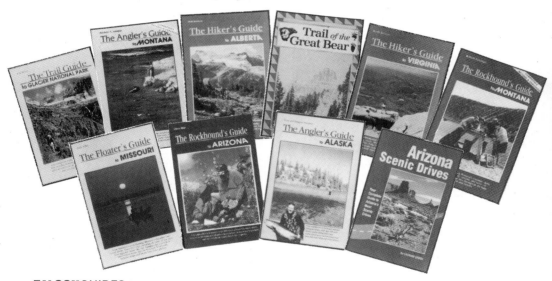

FALCONGUIDES is a series of recreation guidebooks designed to help you safely enjoy the great outdoors. Each title features up-to-date maps, photos, and detailed information on access, hazards, side trips, special attractions, and more. The 6 x 9" softcover format makes every book an ideal travel companion as you discover the scenic wonders around you.

    FALCONGUIDES... leading the way!